Everything you need to know to help you beat cancer

By Chris Woollams MA (Oxon)

Second Edition: February 2003

First Published in June 2002 by:
Health Issues Ltd
The Elms, Radclive Road, Gawcott, Buckingham, MK18 4JB.
Tel: 01280 815166
Fax: 01280 824655
Email: enquiries@iconmag.co.uk

Revised and reprinted February 2003

Cover design by Jeremy Baker.

ISBN 0-9542968-0-X

Printed in England by Bath Press Ltd, Lower Bristol Road, Bath, BA2 3BL

For Catherine

'It is under the greatest adversity that there exists the greatest potential for doing good, both for oneself and others.'

Tenzin Gyatso,
His Holiness the fourteenth Dalai Lama

<u>Important Notice</u>

This book represents a précis of a vast number of varied sources available to anyone on the subject of cancer, its prevention and cure.

Whilst the author has made every effort to ensure that the facts, information and conclusions are accurate and as up to date as possible at the time of publication, the author and publisher assume no responsibility for errors, omissions, or their consequences.

The author is neither a fully qualified health practitioner nor a doctor of medicine, and so is not qualified to give any advice on any medical matters. Cancer (and its related illnesses) is a very serious and very individual disease. Readers must consult with experts and specialists in the appropriate medical field before taking, or refraining from taking, any action.

This book, and the advice contained, is not intended as an alternative to such specialist advice, which should be sought for accurate diagnosis and before any course of treatment.

The author and the publisher cannot be held responsible for any actions that are taken by any reader as a result of information contained in the text of this book. Such action is taken entirely at the reader's own risk.

Author's Note

This book is the second edition of *Everything you need to know to help you beat cancer*. The first run sold out in less than five months, making it probably the fastest selling cancer book in the UK of all time. All the more remarkable, when you realise that the impetus was generated almost entirely through word of mouth. The phone calls, letters and emails have been wonderful. *'Positive'*, *'informative'*, *'easy to read and understand'*, *'inspirational'*, *'down to earth'*, *'practical'*; a phenomenal response from people living with cancer, those who want to prevent it, doctors, nurses, carers, indeed everybody. Thank you.

This new edition contains almost 300 new paragraphs containing up-to-date information on cancer prevention and 'cure'. It is our intention to revise the book every year. So that *Everything you need to know to help you beat cancer* is always the single fount of knowledge it was intended to be, and truly becomes a 'bible' for anyone wishing to prevent or attempt to beat cancer.

The monthly magazine *Integrated Cancer and Oncology News* (ICON), is also thriving. It brings up to the minute information, articles and stories to people touched by cancer, doctors, nurses, carers and those who simply want to prevent it.

What started as a book has become a mission. The website www.iconmag.co.uk should be the first port of call for anyone interested in cancer. It also lists my (now international) speaking venues. Over the next 12 months several new books will be launched, one on specific cancers and ways to try to beat them; plus another on foods, meal preparation and recipes, in conjunction with a famous chef.

And to think I was happily retired!

CONTENTS

VI.   You really can beat cancer – a summary

FOREWORD

By Dr Diane Keith – a practising general practitioner

There have been many, too many times in the last 20 years, when I have sat in my surgery preparing to tell a patient that they have cancer. It's a disease which occurs with increasing frequency and must be considered of epidemic proportions.

I have to steel myself against the patient's inevitable reaction, when they realise that now, more than ever, they will need a great deal of support.

Obviously my job is to help provide some of that support in whatever way I can, to explain treatments and options, to discuss them all thoroughly, and always, always to give hope.

This is where this excellent book will help patients, their families and doctors alike. It is a mass of widely researched information and jammed full of helpful tips. Frankly, it was a real eye-opener to read just how much is known about cancer and the ways of overcoming it.

Crucially, it can also help non-sufferers; people who are currently healthy and do not want to become merely part of the growing statistics.

This book sets out to provide a simple summary of all the basic information and knowledge you require at your fingertips. It is deliberately written in plain English. And that is just what we all need.

The old expression, never give up, is so true when it comes to the lot of the cancer sufferer, their family, and friends. And this book makes you realise just how much is actually known and available, to make us all feel more optimistic.

It also clarifies one important point: that cancer need not be inevitable, bad luck, or something that runs in the family. With a little effort and sensible self-discipline it can very likely be prevented in the first place.

This book is extensive in its coverage and does not pretend to go into vast detail nor baffle with science. Re-read a chapter again and, if you are not sure about something, go and talk to your GP. Take the book with you.

I commend this book as a valuable extra weapon to all those who want to beat cancer.

I now have something very positive to put into my patients' hands, and I for one, am thankful.

Dr Diane Keith, Surrey, England. June 2002.

PREFACE

Over the next few days as you read this book at your leisure, you will come to realise just how much is actually known about cancer; its causes and prevention, its origins and its possible cures.

Depending upon our age, diet and lifestyle, our bodies make between 200 and 1,000 cancer or pre-cancerous cells every day. The statistics show that a cancer will affect one in three of us, and one in four of those affected will die.

But look at these figures another way. Despite producing cancer cells day in, day out, two thirds of us will never contract the disease and, of those who do, 75 per cent will beat it!

Why? Because each of us is a wonderfully tuned and self-protecting living organism, improved and perfected over millions of years to survive most of the harmful things the universe throws our way.

That protection is provided by our **immune system**, the two most important words you need to know when it comes to this subject. You should learn to love your immune system, to nurture it, and maximise it, because you need it in tip-top condition every minute, of every hour, of every day you live. And there are many, many things you can do to strengthen it, just as there are all too many things that you do already that weaken it.

Whilst I do have a strong conviction that cancer is beatable, you need to accept that it occurs through a complex multi-stage process. Beating it is equally a multi-stage task – as individual as each of us is individual. Furthermore, there is no one disease called cancer, any more than there is one form of influenza or one type of cold. Cancer is a generic term for a similar but very individual group of diseases. So this book makes no claims, and offers no promises.

What is clear, is that being healthy cannot be simply regarded as ensuring all your mechanical parts are in working order. Your health stems from your attitude to life, your body's energy systems, endocrine, blood, and lymph systems, well ahead of any problem in a localised area such as your breast or prostate. So when you read the sections on diet, exercise, and supplements understand this: whilst these areas are crucial to your health, so is your overall happiness, your sense of purpose, the laughter you share with friends and even your sex life. All these things can and do affect your immune system.

A healthy life is about balance. Think of it as a health bank balance. There are constant and increasing drains on your resources, large debits every time you drink too much, smoke or become stressed. But you can cut some of those bills if you want to. You can also do a lot to increase the credit side of your health bank balance as you will see in the sections that follow.

The first aim of this book is to save you time and effort, and to provide you with a complete summary of everything I have learned whilst trying to help my daughter with her cancer. I've scoured books and research papers, informed articles and the internet, talked to oncologists (cancer specialists), doctors and alternative health experts.

The second aim is to write a simple book that could not only be read in just a few days, but with a format that would make it a simple reference guide to be returned to, depending upon your specific needs. Whilst the book has breadth, it certainly is not a text book, nor did I want to go too deeply into often complex detail. Of course there is more to find out, more to learn. And because things are changing all the time, I've included a further reading list, helpful phone numbers and internet sites should you want to find out more. *Icon* magazine will help you in this as will our web site (www.iconmag.co.uk).

This book is a précis of the vast amount of information received. Where possible I have tried to highlight both sides of an argument.

I am a biochemist and deal in facts about what affects the cell, its systems, or indeed the whole body. I am not interested in the petty squabbles between individuals in the medical profession and individuals in alternative medicine. Cancer is a serious subject and solutions must be all-embracing, covering everything from surgery to supplements and from radiotherapy to reiki.

Eliminating the cancer tumour rather than the root cause, runs the risk of it returning in the longer term. What good does chopping it out do, if the patient persists with some behaviour that actually caused the original problem, like smoking? True, you buy time with which to analyse the possible causes and ideally correct the underlying problem. But do the patients and the medical profession use that time searching out the causes, the toxins and the lifestyle factors?

Sadly, a lack of time forces too many doctors to focus on the localised cancer and not the whole patient. Is this why we see only three out of several hundred cancers where there are full medical cures and why doctors, instead, talk about remission or extending the active life of sufferers? Certainly no one should blame the doctors; they are paid to be experts in surgery, or radiotherapy or chemotherapy. And that's exactly what they are. Indeed they can qualify as doctors without spending a single day learning about nutrition, biochemistry or body energy.

Having explored the topic pretty comprehensively, my conclusion is simple. Most cancers are beatable. There is simply no need to be a statistic in this epidemic if you know what to do, and then take action.

What is clear to me is that we all have to re-educate ourselves. We need to realise that across a vast expanse of time we developed an interdependent and symbiotic relationship with our environment. After millions of years of slow and even negligible change, the last 150 years have produced dramatic changes in our environment and dangers for all of us. As individuals, we need to learn the science of cancer prevention.

Every government works on the straight-line principle; namely that next year will be better than this, and the year after better than the last. Recessions are but mere blips in a continuous upward trend. Any biologist will tell you that life just is not like that. All life is cyclical. As populations of animals increase, for example lemmings, they become out of balance with their environment and this in turn provides a restricting and self-limiting control on the population. We might worry about specific problems like nuclear power and possible mishaps, but we give little thought to a lifestyle that involves extensive use of, say, cars and computers, farmed food, and chemical toxins. A sedentary lifestyle, for example, coupled with increasing consumption of fats from farmed animals and fish will ultimately weaken our immune systems. Coupled with other environmentally negative influences, it is highly likely this will 'self regulate' our population. We may be talking decades rather than years, but what will the educated populations think when life expectancy rates start to fall?

Meanwhile those same governments aided by the drug companies and charities spend truly vast sums of money on cancer 'cures'. In the year 2000 in the USA those combined forces spent $11bn. Compared to this, the amount spent on cancer prevention was negligible, less than 1 per cent. Phrases like, 'locking the stable door after the horse has bolted', spring to mind.

Within this worsening big picture, it is quite possible for you to create your own highly successful micro-environment and this book will help you. Getting back to basics is an important start. The basis of cancer prevention is common sense. Try to cut the unnecessary toxins out of your life and add back in the things that will boost your immune system to its maximum. Vote with your feet and your wallet.

The great majority of cancer sufferers are not victims. Few are unlucky and catch it from some passing stranger by viral infection, which directly causes cancer. Prevention is in your own hands. And cure is available for almost everybody who is prepared to be positive, more open-minded and more all embracing of the knowledge and facts that exist.

Finally I'd like to say a personal thank you to the people who helped with this book, or should I say mission! Dr Diane Keith, Larry Brooks, Richard Waters, Marie Pay and especially to Lindsey Fealey and my editor Sian Carter. Your comments and help were invaluable.

Chris Woollams
February 2003

INTRODUCTION
Catherine

My daughter Catherine is 24 years old, happy, fun loving, good looking and clever. A couple of years ago she had just finished a chemistry and law degree at Bristol University. She also had cancer.

Over the weekend of the 21 April 2001 we were celebrating my second daughter's 18th birthday with a Saturday dinner, and a Sunday lunch, so the headache on Monday morning was not entirely unexpected, although the sickness was. By Tuesday evening St Thomas' Hospital in London, had given her a scan and we were told Catherine had a brain tumour.

The health system went into overdrive and I have nothing but praise. Catherine was transferred to Queen Square in London to the National Hospital for Neurology, and we were told she would be operated on the following Saturday. No words can express how rapidly your life can change, how the happiness of a birthday weekend could be followed by the crushing horror, fear and sadness of a life-threatening operation.

The excellent surgeon, Mr Kitchen, came out of theatre to tell me that, 'the operation went without incident; (no emotional extremist can presumably even apply to be a brain surgeon). And Catherine seemed to heal by the second during the five days that followed. We were told that small brain tumours were not uncommon; that they had taken most but not all out and with Catherine's age and health, there was little to worry about.

The following Friday we were told what remained of the tumour was malignant.

———————

My personal background includes four years at Oxford University reading biochemistry, with a year specialising in cancer research and viruses. Although I was asked to stay on for a doctorate in cancer research, I am afraid the call of capitalism *was too strong and I spent the next 22 years in advertising and marketing, in the end building a group of nine companies which we put on the stock market. Then I retired aged 45.*

Actually I say retired, but it is not a word that really figures in my personal vocabulary. Over the next five or six years I'd helped some friends launch companies, but my real interest had been a personal quest to understand what things really make a person healthy.

So I read and read, primarily about nutrition, but that spun off into an interest in anti-ageing and body energy systems. Just for fun I did a reiki course and even became a personal trainer, and my business experience helped to launch two health clubs for Virgin.

When Catherine was first diagnosed I did what any good father, biochemist and marketing man would do. I did my home-work. I rang experts in the USA, the UK, and France, gleaned information and second opinions from medical and alternative experts, read so many books we could have opened our own health library, and became a regular on the internet.

I came to three crucial conclusions:

*Firstly, **all the information does exist, if you have the time and the inclination to look.** Sadly there seems to be no single definitive and detailed guide to the prevention or cure of cancer. No easy to read 'fount of knowledge'. Nor do scientists in general seem to be passing the information on to the patient or their local GP or specialist.*

*Secondly, the sad fact is that **people are dying of ignorance. Knowledge is power. And with cancer, knowledge can be the difference between life and death.** Moreover, the onus for managing the solution and all its elements, lies with you the patient.*

*Thirdly, **do everything in your power not to get cancer in the first place.** Spending some time and effort adopting a new lifestyle with the help of this book will give you an invaluable insurance policy in terms of prevention. And my main piece of advice is: 'Love your immune system'!*

Catherine had lots of questions that deserved and demanded definitive, factual answers. And so we come to this book. I hunted high and low to get answers. The problem for most people is that they simply do not have the time to read hundreds of books, articles and look at internet sites, especially if they are suffering from cancer. Worse, some of the books need a biochemist to understand them, whilst others are too simplistic, and most only cover a part of the information available. Some are very personal and relate to an individual cancer, and all too many deteriorate into a glorified recipe book without the glossy photographs.

The great majority also seem to dwell on the problems and the morbid statistics in their opening chapters. This just puts the cancer sufferer off the book. As Catherine said to me: "Dad, I'm not interested in cancer. I'm interested in living!"

Catherine was asking questions that went right across the disease from A to Z, and although we did find all the answers we wanted, we simply couldn't find them in one place.

But then came the defining moment: the real raison d'être for my pieces of paper to come together in a 'Cancer Prevention and Cure Bible'.

Catherine and I were with her oncologist discussing her radio-therapy some four weeks into the six week course. He had already informed her that her chances of surviving five years were approximately 15 per cent, so we knew the seriousness of the situation.

I asked him one straightforward question, 'Exactly what supplements would you give Catherine to improve her chances and the radiotherapy's performance?' To which he replied, 'Well you're the biochemist, you'd know better than me!'.

Saying that I wanted to give her a detox, he replied, 'I don't know what you mean by detox – if you mean antioxidants I'm against them because I read in the paper that they give them to astronauts to prevent the negative effect of radiation in space. But I want the radiation to work'. I interjected that, "Vitamin E would not some-how mystically shield a cancer cell but promote the immune system and selenium .....". He cut me off to say that they had conducted tests and shown that selenium supplements improved the effective-ness of radiotherapy, as did soya isoflavones.

3

All I could say was, 'When did you intend to tell us this?' and vow to myself that I'd write down all my research findings in a single source, in plain simple English, with no complex and baffling scientific or medical jargon, for everybody's benefit. Fortunately, we already had Catherine on selenium and isoflavones, but if I hadn't been a biochemist or done my home-work how would we have known?

Perhaps I'm being a bit naughty here. In my view Catherine would not have survived without surgery, radiotherapy and the excellence of her doctors. And the doctors are trained to think in terms of best practice, which means that they are not encouraged to think 'outside of the box'. Their training leads them to pre-scribe things that have gone through a system of rigorous testing. Selenium and isoflavones haven't had proper clinical trials completed and without published data, doctors are not in a posi-tion to make hard and fast recommendations. If there is a fault, it clearly lies in the system not the people working in it.

With Catherine I became her manager and the 'nag', ringing her up about diet, chasing her with supplements, encouraging her into yoga, sending her to cranial osteopaths, and arranging trips to shows and events to maintain her positive attitude. We even planned to launch a monthly cancer help magazine, which is not only much needed but could give her a sense of purpose.

I am pleased to say this project reached fruition with the launch of Icon *(Integrated Cancer and Oncology News) in July 2002.*

It has been a great success, and is a way of keeping people up-to-date with all the latest news as well as sharing their ideas and experiences. We have also launched our website www.iconmag.co.uk which we hope will be the first port of call for anyone interested in beating cancer. Again it is in the same style: an 'integrated' approach to cancer, informative and inspirational.

If you are unfortunate enough to contract cancer you have to muster every armament you can to aid your fire-power and rid yourself of it. You need to go to an oncologist who is experienced in your type of cancer, who is fighting alongside you and provid-ing you with lots of useful information. A friend whose daughter had skin cancer said her specialist gave her computer printouts and photostats an inch thick so that she could be fully informed. Don't settle for less. Ask and be pushy because the standards of support vary so much between specialists. If you are going to homeopaths, cranial osteopaths or healers, go to experts on your type of cancer. Get second and third opinions from people with recent experience, and check and double-check their opinions and recommendations.

Someone has to manage and co-ordinate the multitude of treatments available. The cancer patients themselves will become depressed, through circumstance, or treatment or both, and a friend or relative must take on the role of minder (even though I'm sure Catherine wished I'd go away on many occasions).

Finally though, I believe beating cancer is about odds and, particularly, improving your odds. **If you get cancer you do not want to be the average case.**

With Catherine we have done everything in our power to increase the odds in her favour.

Through Western diet, being overweight, smoking, drinking, and pollution, the odds on you contracting cancer are increasing, if you just go with the flow.

As Samuel Johnson said, 'The chains of habit are too weak to be felt until they are too strong to be broken'. With the modern world dragging you into bad habits, only serious self-discipline will get you out of becoming more and more at risk.

There is no doubt that at university Catherine had fallen into bad habits. These, coupled with an ongoing illness that was never adequately addressed, worsened her odds to the point where a cancer developed.

We believe we have learned what caused her cancer and what was sustaining it. This aligned with some excellent modern medical care, numerous 'complementary health' treatments and a whole re-education process on her diet and lifestyle, have increased Catherine's odds for survival. Catherine herself has been absolutely brilliant and completely reinvented herself in terms of diet, lifestyle, exercise, and attitude. Above all, her determination and the wonderful support of her friends (and she has many) helped this enormously.

5

But this book is actually for people who want to prevent the onset of cancer just as much as it is for those with cancer. In both cases increasing the odds is about knowing the facts and understanding likely causes and likely solutions. The self-discipline needed simply needs to be even more rigorous if you have already contracted cancer.

So I pass on my answers to Catherine's questions to anybody who wants to read them. I hate to think that a lack of information or worse, misinformation, would result in any more unnecessary deaths when so much hard evidence is available, if only one knew where to start looking.

No one wants cancer. Now I've seen it first hand I can assure you it is a dreadful problem to have. Everybody should do everything in their power to prevent themselves from getting it.

Hopefully this book is a good place to start.

SECTION I

A guide to cancer in
plain English

Q1. What is cancer?

A cancer tumour starts with an initial rogue cell. If it beats your body's defence systems it behaves like a foetal cell dividing and copying itself very rapidly but in an uncontrolled manner. Since such cells can divide as often as once every 20 minutes, the original rogue cell can grow into a core malignant tumour very quickly.

A tumour is an unusual growth in the body. Some tumours are benign (ie grow at only a modest rate and do not spread); whilst some are malignant (ie grow rapidly and do spread within that tissue or to other parts of the body). This malignancy is what is commonly described as cancer.

Cells from the core tumour can also break away acting as 'negative disciples' sending out the havoc message to other places in the body (metastasis). When this message reaches another cell in another part of the body, it can enter that cell and turn it rogue too.

The original tumour is called the primary, the new tumours in other parts of the body are called secondaries. Some tumours, for example primary brain tumours, are confined to such tight spaces that they have difficulty sending out rogue messages. More often though, tumours, for example breast tumours, not only send out the rogue message to places like the liver or brain where they can initiate secondaries, but often the rogue messengers collect in the lymph nodes. This is because of the action of the body's immune defence system which has carted off a couple of rogue cells to the lymph nodes in order to study them and try to produce a neutralising antibody. The rogue cancer cells actually collect in and 'poison' the very cells that are trying to eradicate them (this will be explained in far more detail in Section II).

Even in normal healthy people several hundred initial rogue cancer and pre-cancer cells are made every day, but these are rendered harmless through the body's various immune defence systems.

So there are three opportunities to control cancer: neutralizing the rogue cells; stopping tumour growth; preventing the rogue cells from spreading.

Q2. What makes a cancer cell?

A number of degenerative diseases are thought to be caused by a 'triple whammy' and cancer almost certainly arises in the same way.

Firstly, you have to have some genetic predisposition or weakness. In the case of cancer, this is probably inherent in nearly all of us.

If you take people from China or Japan, where certain cancers hardly exist, and subject them to Western pollution, diet and lifestyle, their rates of cancer increase in line with the native inhabitants. However, it has been estimated from research studies that only 10 per cent of all cancers can be solely attributed to genetic defects. Even if cancer runs in your family there is a great deal you can do to avoid it, and your chances of success with the right tactics are high.

Secondly, you need a negative environment around the cell.

This can be caused by tobacco, sunlight, pesticides, diet, in fact a whole host of things including stress. In one region of Africa the bite of a fly causes the weakness.

Every one of us has an immune system, our natural defence against foreign invaders like viruses. This system will usually recognise a rogue cell or its message and attempt to neutralise it. In a healthy body under normal conditions, rogue cells are mopped up all the time. But, the effects of a poor diet, pesticides, smoking, alcohol, excess fats, and age, weaken the immune system. Sometimes it is stretched to breaking point dealing with the production of rogue cells.

Thirdly, you need 'the final straw', something to tip your biological balance over the edge.

If, for example, on top of everything else the body gets an infection, which further weakens the immune system, the rogue cells will start to win their battle. Since the immune system weakens markedly with age, for reasons we will explore later, this 'triple whammy' is most often seen with older people. But not always.

The idea that you need all three factors explains why some diseases (eg heart problems, high cholesterol) run in families, yet some members can and do avoid them. But they avoid them by not falling into the same traps as their other family members, for example, by watching their diet or taking exercise. Recent research on inherited diseases in Scandinavia using twins supports this totally. The *New England Journal of Medicine* reports on 4,788 pairs of twins from Scandinavia who were studied, and concluded that, 'Inherited genetic factors make a minor contribution to the susceptibility of most types of cancer'. The USA National Cancer Institute said, 'This study should dispel the fatalism of the general public that if it runs in my family, I'm doomed'.

Cancer, like heart disease, can be avoided and beaten if you take positive action and work at it.

It demands effort and discipline in a world that is actively and increasingly working against you. Make no mistake, there are many things you can do to prevent or stop cancer.

The Chinese have a saying, 'Treating a person when they become ill is like starting to dig a well when you are thirsty.'

From the cancer patients I have seen and talked to, I counsel everyone to do everything in their power to avoid getting cancer in the first place. And to cancer sufferers I would say, 'Think very seriously about what diet, lifestyle and psychological problems might have caused the cancer and work hard to undo the damage.' You can do it if you really want to.

Q3. How does a cancer cell develop?

Every cell in your body has a nucleus, the 'control centre' for your whole body and your whole life. Inside it is your DNA, which I want you to imagine as a very, very long but infinitesimally fine string wrapped up in a tight ball.

Along the length of this DNA string is a code made up of a sequence of chromosomes unique to you. This is your personal blueprint, and it sends out messages telling your body to make five fingers, two legs, blue eyes and blond hair. The ball is loosely 'glued' together by histamines and other substances. Some parts of the ball of string are exposed to the outside world, other parts are not.

Inside the nucleus you also have substances which work like little trains. On the string there are little 'start' points and little 'stop' points.

The trains see a start point, jump on and go along the string until they hit a stop point. They then fall off. The code in between the start and stop is read by the train, which copies it and sends the exact copy off as a message to the world outside the nucleus. Obviously the trains can only read a full sequence if it is exposed and not buried deep inside the ball.

Imagine that one day the effect of your lifestyle, diet, and an infection all cause the ball of string to be surrounded by toxins, which have found their way into the nucleus and the fluid around the ball of string. The toxins may attack the string and even unravel it slightly. Other bits of code are suddenly freed to be read, and other start and stop points are seen by the train. So it reads them and sends out new messages.

Almost all of these messages may be gobbledegook and mean nothing to the systems around the body reading them. The body's immune system simply rejects and neutralises them rendering them harmless. Others though can be rogue cancer precursors.

In fact you need to imagine our ball as having two parts, a red part and a smaller blue part. The blue part itself actually has an in-built defence system to recognise the rogue messages first and order the body to neutralise them.

Some may get past this blue defence system, but the healthy

body has a second line of defence, a strong immune system, which is ready for these 'escapees' and mops them up.

Real problems come when a cancer message has been produced by our trains; or a mistake happens in the blue part, the part that is there to defend you; or if the outer body is not healthy and the immune defence system is weak.

There are a number of ways in which the original messages can be rogue. Sometimes chromosomes stick together, sometimes a bit breaks off. Sometimes bits become reassembled in the wrong order. Rarely, too, the DNA isn't copied perfectly when the original cell divides to make new ones, so an ABCDE code becomes ABXDE.

The point is that whatever the particular detailed explanation of a rogue message, it is invariably formed by the DNA string ball being bathed in toxins inside the nucleus.

These toxins or poisons cause the attack on the ball of string and the malfunctioning and misreading to take place.

All remains manageable as long as both the blue defence system in the DNA string works and the overall immune system is strong. But what happens when the actual piece of DNA that is your front line defender is the piece that is poisoned, and it is the blue part that sends out a cancer message?

Up to half of all cancers are thought to be caused by the 'defender' portion of the DNA itself going wrong. Smoking, UV light, asbestos and many more substances can cause this.

In this case a rogue message breaks out with no 'front line' DNA defence to stop it and, if it beats the more general immune system too, becomes a cancer cell, then a cancer tumour.

When a tumour gets to a size of about one centimetre it also needs a blood supply, and it is at this time it starts to grow unchecked. Restricting the growth of the specific blood supply is also an opportunity in our attempt to control cancer.

The fact that this is a complex multi-step process (in fact far more complex than I have actually described) makes it all the more likely that only rarely does only one toxin cause the problem. This is why people with several 'problems', for example, poor environment, poor diet, smoking and alcohol, significantly worsen their odds. Again, everyone of us should recognise this fact.

Q4. How does my DNA become 'poisoned'?

Imagine your cell looking like a poached egg in a pot of water. The yolk is the nucleus, inside which sits your ball of string, the DNA bathed in fluid. In the white of the egg, the cellular liquid, are lots of little power stations called mitochondria, which burn sugar by a process called the Krebs cycle to provide energy for the cell to function. Surrounding the cell, our whole egg, is water or 'lymph'. Beyond the water is the blood system with blood flowing within a more structured tube like system. Each element of this cellular, lymph and blood system is separated from the next by a membrane largely made up of protein and fats.

Day in, day out, the power stations burn fuel and oxygen to make energy, and waste products are produced. Proteins and fats come into the cell because they are needed to rebuild the cellular structures, like the DNA string itself or the membranes. All these nutrients pass from the blood to the lymph to the cellular liquid (the cytoplasm) and some into the nucleus.

So our ball of string ends up surrounded by a fluid in which there are waste products and inbound nutrients. Worse, some irregular fuels cause the power stations to emit nasty black smoke, which makes the whole environment in there very unpleasant. Some inbound substances also have a polluting effect on our egg yolk.

Also, some of the things coming from the blood system via the lymph may not be nutrients but may themselves be pollutants; for example, the byproducts of smoking, or drinking alcohol.

The nastiest pollutants are called free radicals, and their action is to change the molecules they bump into, in the same way that air turns a half-eaten apple brown. This process is called oxidation. They do this because they are incomplete and have a loose, sticky end, which rips parts off other molecules. These damaged molecules in turn can attack others, starting an ongoing chain reaction.

Free radicals are aggressive and they may well stick to our DNA string causing it to change structurally, blocking accurate

DNA replication. It should be noted that there is some evidence that taking iron supplements actually heightens this aggression and, for example, many anti-ageists steer clear of supplements containing iron.

The crucial point is that you can make your egg white and egg yolk more polluted by, for example, what you burn at the power stations; or by having stagnant, polluted surrounding lymph. If your blood is carrying more toxins, so too will be your lymph and then your cell. So the DNA string is increasingly surrounded by

- More cell produced toxins
- More 'ingested' toxins.

The body does have a double protection system for mopping up free radicals (as we will see in more detail later) namely

- Antioxidants
- Hormones.

Both of these specifically neutralise free radicals. But, especially as you age, the flow of lymph past the cell is reduced resulting in more waste build-up, and the level of hormones acting to neutralise free radicals decreases.

(You may remember from your school days that you can take a beaker of blue liquid, separate it from a beaker of clean water by a membrane or filter paper and, after a reasonable period of time, half the blue will go across into the original jar of clean water. It's called osmosis and happens until the liquid on the two sides of the filter membrane is at the same concentration. Well, that is pretty much how the waste moves out of the egg yolk (the nucleus) into the white (the cell) and into the watery lymph.

In your school experiment, if you wanted more of the blue to go you had to keep changing the beaker of clean water. So too with lymph. It needs to be clean and flowing to take away the maximum amount of waste. If it is not, then the DNA string in our nucleus may, before too long, be swimming in very polluted and toxic fluid.)

In summary

- Do not ingest unnecessary extra toxins
- Keep your lymph clean and flowing (eg by drinking lots of water and by your own 'movement' which we will explain in Q5)
- Keep your level of antioxidants and hormones up, especially as you age
- Do not over-stress your cellular biochemistry by making the power stations produce excess waste.

With regard to the last point, it is not just the case that burning nasty fuels can over pollute a cell; both an excess of stress hormones or exercising too strenuously will encourage the power stations to work at inefficient levels and produce excess waste.

Cancer cells are different

The poisoning of your cells renders them different in several ways.

When a foetus develops in the womb it starts with one fused cell, and doubles and doubles. Each of these early cells can go on to become an eye cell, or a brain cell or a finger cell. These early cells are called 'stem cells', and they reproduce very, very rapidly until around day 46, when the whole process is hit by a control switch and calms down. At this point all the basic human features have been put in place and a 'normal' growth rate can now take over.

The 'switching off process' is probably controlled by messages from the pancreas (see Q24).

Cancer cells resemble stem cells in that they divide very rapidly, and unlike the defined breast or prostate cells around them, they are still in an undefined and elementary state.

Some parts of the DNA string are also found outside the nucleus and within the mitochondria. The power stations, or mitochondria, in a cancer cell are also very different from those in normal cells.

Under normal conditions oxygen and sugars are used by mitochondria to generate energy. In a cancer cell, oxygen is not used.

17

In fact cancer cells hate oxygen. Energy is made by a different process and the waste product of a cancer cell is lactic acid, the same substance that causes cramp in sportsmen.

Lactic acid is highly toxic, so the surrounding cells are poisoned. The liver is also overworked trying to neutralise this lactic acid.

This may all seem a little complicated but it provides further lessons:

- Keep your system 'oxygenated' through exercise, deep breathing, clean air
- Keep your system moving
- Keep your liver healthy.

Q5. How can I reduce the effect of toxins?

Even if you ate only organic food, used only non-toxic toiletries, drank only the purest water, never touched red meat or dairy products, never smoked or drank alcohol and lived the purest of lives, you would still build up toxins in your body. A number of eminent cancer experts feel that over time it is inevitable that high levels of toxic wastes build up in and around the cell, and this accounts for the fact that 80 per cent of cancers occur in the over 60 age group.

But it is not inevitable.

Move your lymph

As we have said, toxins inside the cell move into the liquid outside the cell (the lymph) and are taken away. The lymph then passes them into the blood system which takes it via the liver and kidneys to be excreted. So the lymph plays a crucial role in keeping your cells toxin free.

However, unlike the blood system where the action of the heart keeps it moving, the lymph, which has twice the total volume of the blood in your body, has little or nothing to keep it flowing – except for your own activity.

If you are dehydrated or inactive you will build up more toxins around your cells.

Activities like t'ai chi, or aerobic exercise (which encourages the pumping of the blood and in turn massages the lymph system into action) move the toxins out. But this only does part of the job. The most important thing to do every day is to open up your chest by moving your arms wide. This is because the largest channel of lymph, called the thoracic duct, lies across the chest and stimulating movement of this is crucial to good lymph flow.

Swimming is excellent, especially the breaststroke. Press-ups are also good. Certain yoga exercises, like the salutation to the sun, the cobra and the shoulder stand, really get the thoracic lymph moving. Even laughing deeply massages the thoracic duct, as does deep breathing (which is an important aspect of yoga).

Sleep also aids lymph movement, because when you are horizontal it does not have to fight gravity. Conversely, people who don't stand up straight risk restricting their thoracic lymph flow.

Massage, particularly deep massage such as Thai massage or shiatsu, stimulates the lymph system and gets it moving. The term lymphatic drainage is often correctly applied to this form of massage.

Detoxification and fibre

Regular bowel movements and a clean liver also help to detoxify the cellular system. Everybody should ensure they have:

• A good intake of fibre from plants, vegetables and fruits (psyllium seeds are a good addition to breakfast cereals).

A diet high in fibre is directly linked to reduced body toxins and high fibre in the colon helps carry more toxins and, for example, excess hormones out of the body. But it is not just in the bowels that fibre does its work. Phytates and lignans, two commonly occurring substances in plant fibre, stick to the free radicals and neutralise them, like the actions of antioxidants beta-carotene and lycopene. Which is why diet is so important in reducing the toxic waste in and around cells.

• A good intake of water throughout the day, especially after exercise or massage.

This is essential to flush toxins out of the blood and lymph. The accepted view is that you should drink at least 1.5 litres per day but an eminent bottled water company admitted to me that there is no research to support this. It is felt by many medical practitioners that many of us are dehydrated and there is a lot of justification in encouraging all of us to consume at least 1.5 litres per day (but not with meals as it dilutes the enzymes needed for proper food digestion).

• A detox once per month for at least three to four days.

The issue of detoxing produces heated debate in some medical quarters but users feel strongly about the benefits. The whole area of juice diets and detoxing will be covered later in the book.

Boost your natural defences

The biggest neutraliser of the toxins and free radicals is the immune system aided and abetted by the endocrine system.

Taking beta-carotene, vitamin C and vitamin E, for example, boosts the neutralising ability of the immune system.

Hormones such as growth hormone, melatonin and DHEA also significantly help to 'mop up' free radicals as do a number of co-factors like coenzyme Q10 (CoQ10) – all will be covered in more detail in question 18. Unfortunately all the latter four 'good guys' peak in the body between the ages of 16–20 and then steadily decrease to the point of almost non-existence by the age of 70. This is a crucial reason for excess toxic waste in old people.

The good news is you can do something about this. For example, experiments with people over 60 taking 60 mgs per day of CoQ10 for three months returned them to levels found in 20 year olds. We shall see later that you can take action to keep your hormone levels as high as possible as you age.

Having a slightly alkaline body (in a world where most of us have an acid body) is essential to the proper working of the immune system.

Omega 3 has a huge effect on detoxing the cellular surroundings, as does providing a good supply of oxygen.

Acidophilus and other 'friendly' bacteria in your gut are your first line of defence, and recent research even suggests that pieces of their cell walls can kill cancer cells in vitro tests.

Q6. Are overweight people more prone to cancer?

In early 2003 researchers at the Erasmus Medical Centre in Rotterdam re-analysed an American study involving 3,457 participants aged 30 to 49 and followed over a 42 year period. The results were reported in the *Annals of Internal Medicine*. They concluded that:
- 40 year old male and female non-smokers who were 4–10 kgs over a healthy weight lost 3 years off their life expectancy.
- When the excess exceeded 12 kgs women lost 7 years and men 5.8.
- If they smoked as well, these figures became a loss of 13.5 years.

Another study concluded that overweight and obese people are 40 per cent more likely to contract cancer and it is quite easy to see why.

If you eat more, quite simply, you produce more toxic waste products.

If you are overweight you are probably less active, your lymph system stagnates and so the toxins stay in the cellular environment longer.

Often overweight people are overweight because of the types of food they eat. These foods are often high on the list of 'bad foods'. Poor quality eating habits are formed at an early age.

One third of boys under 6 are overweight or obese, rising to almost 50 per cent by the age of 15. Fatty foods and empty calories are destroying these humans early. Fats, fizzy drinks, salted and preserved food, processed quick meals, the list is endless. Parents have a duty to bring their kids up properly and at least half are failing them. Almost half of all children eat no vegetables in a week apart from chips! Recent UK research showed that half of the 10 year olds surveyed could not even identify basic vegetables like cauliflower and broccoli. Schools need to educate the next generation that vegetables are red, green, white and orange and rarely come in fast food cartons.

Food is often prepared in a less than beneficial way. Over-weight people are often great 'snackers'. As we shall see, biscuits, crisps and chips are sources of highly carcinogenic acrylamides. Frying uses oils that give rise to free radical toxins; food burnt on the barbecue creates nitrosamines, which are carcinogenic; boiling is normally overdone and the vitamins leave with the boiling water. The moral is to eat raw, steamed and slow roasted foods. Let us even see the return of the old fashioned stew with its vegetables and nourishment values. Parents need to get back to basics in their cooking and provision of foods at home.

Poor eating habits, particularly the consumption of high calorie foods of little nutritional benefit put all people at increased risk of cancer, especially overweight people. The hormones in a healthy body are in a perfect state of balance (homeostasis). Drink lots of fizzy sweet drinks and that all changes instantly because the body produces a surge of insulin to deal with the excess sugar. This then has a knock-on effect to the other hormones in the body and, as we will see in Q19, can nega-tively influence the cellular environment. Overweight people often eat in such a way (eg big meals, high fat meals, lots of sugary foods) that they suddenly flood their bodies with sugar and carbohydrates and these play havoc with their hormones.

And hormones are extremely powerful biochemical substances. A small excess or lack can cause a chain reaction in the body, affecting the immune system and the ability of the body to mop up free radicals, worsening the odds against cancer.

Overweight people also have excess fat stores and fat is a wonderful solvent. It can dissolve, and so hold, more toxins including excess hormones. If an overweight person also fails to encourage lymph movement, the toxins that cannot leave in a dynamic, flowing lymph system will happily be dissolved by the fat cells rendering our fat person extremely toxic, with far higher levels of unwanted hormones, and far more prone to diseases including cancer. A simple case of 'Toxic Waist'!

By contrast, tests on laboratory rats where the calorie count was held at 10 per cent below the normal required daily level, showed 40 per cent increases in life expectancy over the norm.

The evidence is overwhelming.

Q7. How does cancer spread?

The original rogue cell with its unravelled ball of DNA string can simply copy itself repeatedly. And the message to the cellular system is often to do this very rapidly in much the same way as foetal cells divide.

Perfect copies of the new slightly looser ball of string are made from the original, because the body normally does copy perfectly. So suddenly there are many cells all with the new-look ball of string. Theoretically, if the environment of this cell is maintained (eg if the diet, smoking, sunlight conditions continued) the rogue ball of string becomes the norm in an area of the body.

Meanwhile, the great majority of cells in the body are still in their original state, as is your protective immune system. The healthy immune system should recognise the rogue cells and simply kick them out, if it is strong enough to do so. As we will see later, it has identifier T cells that look round the body for rogue cells and then bring out the troops to kick them out.

Cancer spreads because the original rogue cell and any copies are also sending out messages into the rest of the body. Just as the train read the ball of string and sent a message from the nucleus into the cell, another copy is made in the cell and can be sent in the blood stream throughout the body. This secondary message acts very much like virus and it can poison and decode a recipient cell. Some rogue cells spread via the blood system to secondary organs like the brain or the liver; some spread via the lymph to lymph nodes. Metastasis is the name given to this process of spreading, and also to the secondary tumours resulting.

However, the fact that hundreds of such messages can be sent out but usually no recipients are infected, means that your body is normally extremely successful in protecting itself. And the fact that cancer sufferers can go into remission or are cured certainly indicates that the body can, **at any time** 'restrengthen' itself and halt the advances of the rogue cells. This is the power of the immune system.

The issue for everybody is to realise that there are factors that cause cancer and you should do everything in your power to reduce them, whilst also doing everything in your power to boost your immune system. If you are a sufferer already, there are things that are almost certainly 'maintaining' the cancer. You must try to work out what they are because, in the early stages of a cancer, it is quite possible to reduce the negative causes, boost your immune system and stop the tumour in its tracks. I know a homeopath who did exactly that with her own breast cancer.

Cancer does however possess the ability to hide from our immunue system. Not in every case, but sometimes. For example, some tumours can form a 'protein shield' around them making attack very difficult; there are ingredients in a number of natural foods, and there are enzymes that help you break down this coat. In other cancers a particular gene can go wrong on your DNA string. For example, gene BRCA 1 prevents the immune system from recognising the rogue cells. People with this gene need to maintain a very strong immune system.

SECTION II

How can I best protect myself
against cancer?

INTRODUCTION

Sitting at a table out of doors in regional Thailand I ordered grilled fish. It duly arrived complete with an intact liver, a plate of vegetables and a bowl of steamed rice. I was immediately told that eating the liver would make me clever and keep me from being ill. My partner had steamed chicken (although it was a frugal helping by Western standards) cooked in a 'stew' of lemon grass, galanga and kaffir lime leaves.

The next morning the national newspaper reported that cancer rates in Thailand were expected to double from 60,000 per annum to 120,000 in the next 20 years. The reason for this was laid at the door of the West. Fast food and fried chicken restaurants, coffee and muffin shops have arrived. Thais should get back to basics was the cry; more vegetables, fruit and rice.

In my hotel that morning were a hundred or so overweight and unhealthy looking people, mainly Western tourists. Most were tucking into plate upon plate of ham, eggs, cheese, and bread, toasts and croissants, butter and jam. The more healthy minded (I guess) ate muesli and fibre and a low fat yoghurt; while everyone drank tea and coffee, with or without sugar and milk.

The gym was empty.

My Thai partner had a bowl of rice with some chilli and vegetables followed by fresh fruit. Her drink was water.

The population of the UK is approximately the same as that of Thailand. New cancer cases in the UK this year will approach 270,000.

Q8. How likely am I to contract cancer?

Do you get colds or flu? This may seem a little flippant especially as colds or flu are invasions of the body by external viruses, and in cancer something in the very structure of your body has gone wrong. But the action of the rogue cell in sending out messages inside the body is very like the action of a virus; it's just that the origins are from within. With a normal body 'invaded' by 200 plus rogue cells a day, the immune system is called in to play, whether it is a cancer attack or a flu attack. This is why it is important to 'love your immune system'.

Similarly, just as there are many strains of 'cold' or of 'flu', there is no one single cancer. Tumours take many forms, have many starting points and are as individual as you are. Two people diagnosed with the same cancer can have very different causal and biochemical relationships with it. This will affect its growth and their ability to beat it. This is why you do hear such wonderful stories of people 'curing' themselves, whilst others try everything with little success. There is a great deal that every cancer sufferer can do to improve their odds of a cure. There's also a great deal we can all do to prevent a cancer taking hold.

As I said in the introduction, on current statistics two out of three people will not contract cancer. And of cancer sufferers, three quarters will beat it. There are many things you can do to increase the odds, specifically strengthening your immune system and avoiding the pitfalls. As we shall see, you are a complex mixture of hormones, immune and body energy systems, all of which can be boosted to aid your defence. Think positively, be disciplined and realise that, despite the growing worldwide statistics, you can build your own little micro-environment of health. You can increase your odds.

The worldwide statistics on cancer are awesome. It has reached epidemic proportions. After car accidents, leukaemia and brain tumours are the second and third biggest causes of death in children in the Western world. In the next 30 years at least one in eight women will have breast cancer and one in three men over 60 will have prostate cancer. In fact, there are over 200 other forms of cancer including, just for example, lung cancer, skin cancer, stomach and colon cancer, liver and pancreatic cancer.

Four out of 10 people in the UK will get a cancer.

Worse still, the rates are increasing. It is now estimated that, of Americans born today, one in two will develop cancer.

In the UK, childhood cancers are 30 per cent higher than 45 years ago, germ cell tumours are 50 per cent higher, brain cancer is up 36 per cent and acute lymphoblastic leukaemia is up 33 per cent. The odds do not make good reading. If these were road or flying accidents there would be an outcry, a major overhaul on safety and an examination of the causes. Not so with cancer.

As we shall see, certain things you do or use (lifestyle) or eat (diet) can cause a specific problem at any age. But for most people two factors contribute to the fact that 80 per cent of all cancers hit those people over the age of 60:

- **A slow steady build up of toxins as a by-product of our normal daily lives**
- **A natural age related decline in our defensive hormone and immune systems.**

Sir Richard Doll and Sir Richard Peto of Oxford University looked at the causes of cancer in a study funded by the Imperial Cancer Research Fund and the Medical Research Council. They concluded that, for example:

35% cancers were caused		by diet
30%	,,	by smoking
10%	,,	by reproductive hormones
10%	,,	by infection
5%	,,	by alcohol.

They also concluded that only a very small percentage are due to environmental factors or pollution and up to 2 per cent of cancers are caused by some sort of virus, bacterium, parasite or yeast. These figures are likely to be much too small.

If cancer involves a very complex multi-stage process only rarely can it be caused by just one factor, so the above figures seem a bit too black and white to me. Although factors like asbestos and extreme sunshine may cause the whole chain reaction of cancer formation, people are most at risk when hit by several factors, for example, those on a poor diet, who are overweight, smoke, and drink. The odds increase disproportionately the more hits you have.

The above study also seems to fail to fully integrate the role of all environmental factors into this complex process. Clearly air and water impurity, toxin residues in foods, toxins in household products, toiletries and cosmetic products, prescription medicines, and pesticides must all be shaping our overall lives and our health.

To date, the majority of cancers appear to be a more Western lifestyle phenomenon. For instance, breast and prostate cancers are virtually non-existent in China and Thailand, whilst Japan runs at a quarter of the rate in Britain. Even people in Nagasaki and Hiroshima, those sites of nuclear explosions, are only a fifth as likely to get a prostate or breast cancer as people living in the West.

In the 1950s and 60s breast cancer was rare in Japan but the more affluent Japanese women have now forsaken their original, mainly vegetarian rice and vegetable diets to follow a more Western diet of dairy products and meat with alarming consequences. Age adjusted mortality rates in Japan show that in the 30 years from 1968, breast cancer in women and kidney cancer in men have both doubled, whilst kidney cancer in women, brain cancers generally and multiple myeloma have increased by over 300 per cent. The Heidelberg Cancer Research Centre found that vegetarians have more than twice the immune defence ability to knock out cancer cells than non-vegetarians.

Since so few cancers can actually be completely cured by the official medical establishment despite billions of dollars being spent on drug development, the crucial issue is not to contract it in the first place. Published data in the USA shows that apart from major advances in the cure rates of cancers such as testicular and childhood leukaemia, the overall cure rate in the last 10 years is virtually static. In the last 20 years, cure rates increased by barely 10 per cent whilst cancer growth rates increased by 25 per cent or more.

If all this doesn't start a sensible argument for the creation of a serious cancer prevention body there are many hundreds of further facts beyond the scope of this book. Every one of us is vulnerable and we need a good honest appraisal of our lifestyles, our environment, the products we use and our diets.

Where possible a more back to basics approach to living will help, but even that may not be enough with the tide of possible cancer causes flooding our way.

Cancer sufferers often ask themselves: 'Why me?' In fact all non-sufferers should be asking: 'Why not me?'

Q9. What can we learn from cancer sufferers?

When someone has cancer it is a 'must' to look beyond the tumour to the possible causes and elements that are sustaining it. For the sufferer this increases the odds of a cure. But for the non-sufferer it is enormously helpful too. There are generally four factors common to cancer sufferers:

(i) Cancer sufferers are 'toxic', as we have discussed
(ii) Cancer sufferers often have 'acid' bodies
(iii) Cancer sufferers often have a parasite (and/or heavy yeast infection) and about 20 per cent have some sort of virus
(iv) Cancer sufferers often have a self-debilitating mental attitude.

You will note I have not included 'heredity'. This is because of the Swedish research amongst identical twins that I mentioned earlier; that even with similar genes there is much you can do in your diet, attitude, and lifestyle to prevent a cancer occurring. You just have to try harder and take more care!

(i) Toxins

We have already touched on toxins, the need to drink water, take exercise, to avoid certain foods and the need to ensure healthy bowel movements and a clean liver (by, for example, detoxing regularly). We will look at other issues in more detail later.

(ii) Acid bodies

As we have seen, some observers believe 35 per cent of cancers are caused by diet. We will look at the dangers of specific foods, but one observation is made in several books: that cancer sufferers have 'acid bodies'. (Toxins will negatively influence the pH balance of the body making conditions more acid.) However, all foodstuffs can be divided into those that leave an alkaline residue and those that leave an acid one; our modern lifestyle and diet pushes us towards the acid producing foods whereas our fore-fathers 100 years or more ago had an alkaline producing diet.

At a cellular level the biochemical processes **need** a slightly alkaline pH for maximum efficiency and this is essential for the efficacy of the immune system as well.

To beat cancer you must aim to eat less acid producing foods and more alkaline producing foods. That doesn't mean to say you need to stay off the acid producers completely, just be conscious of the two food types and shift your balance more in favour of alkaline producers overall. One thing worth bearing in mind is that acid residue foods tend to be more severe, so you will need

Table I Acid Producers – some examples	
Liver, crab, shellfish,scallops, stress	-5
All meats, lack of sleep, fried foods	-4
Most fish, eggs, crisps, peanuts and similar snacks, processed meats and smoked fish, sauces, vinegars, mustards, chocolate, salt, spirits, white wine, cigarettes.	-3
Most refined wheat based products, fizzy soft drinks, oranges, tomatoes, refined rice, noodles, pasta, coffee, tea, dairy, red wine.	-2
Lentils, chickpeas, dried beans, beer, whole wheat, bananas, prunes, plums.	-1

Table II Alkaline Producers – some examples	
Apples, pears, all green vegetables, cranberries, fresh nuts, melons, pumpkin, onions, oats, millet, rye, asparagus.	+1
All berries, cherries, mangoes, lychees, coconut, peaches, grapes, carrots potatoes, parsnips, turnips, fresh beetroot, lemons, watercress, papaya, whole brown rice, soya beans and soya.	+2
Garlic, kale, dates and figs especially dried, raisins	+3
Cooked spinach, noni juice, fresh ginger.	+4

to consume large quantities of alkaline residue foods just to balance even one or two acid foods.

From various sources I have compiled a gradient of acidity such that acid residue 'beware' is minus 5 points; 'extremely acid' is minus 4 points; 'very acid' minus 3; 'moderately acid' minus 2 and 'slightly acid' minus 1. Alkaline residue producers are given plus points, up to a maximum of 4. (See Tables I and II.)

How well do you do in a day?

As you can see there are not that many high yield alkaline producers. (For a full list of acid and alkaline residue producers, see appendix I.)

You can buy pH testing kits to measure your body's acidity and you can have your blood and cellular biochemistry analysed to check your levels of stress and your vitamin and mineral content.

Often overlooked in the acidity debate is the role of minerals. As we shall discuss later, obtaining adequate supplies of minerals, like calcium, magnesium and some of the essential micro-nutrients, also has a profound alkalising effect on the body. Coral calcium is a strong alkaliser with its organic mineral content.

(iii) Parasites, yeasts, viruses, and bacteria

Parasites
People tend to think of parasites as quite large organisms like tapeworms or liver flukes, but in Carolina over 80 per cent of the population has a parasite. It is microscopic and comes from the water system; it is immune to chlorine. Other microscopic parasites can take up residence having arrived on your fruit.

In one report a doctor in Boston found that 42 of his thousand or so patients had liver fluke and, on killing the parasite, their cancer condition improved markedly. **In another study 80 per cent of cancer patients were found to have a parasite.** Some UK practitioners believe that most, if not all, of their cancer patients have some sort of parasite. Worryingly, since 1997 levels of fluke have quadrupled in British livestock according to government figures.

One reason for the rising incidence of parasites in the USA is felt to be their increased transmission through sexual activity (even simply kissing an infected host). Another is the parasites' diminished requirement for a secondary host in order to survive.

All parasites historically have needed at least two hosts. Now it is felt that certain ingested solvents and pollutants like isopropyl alcohol, a by-product from contaminants of animal fat, pesticides and hygiene products, allow some flukes to multiply in just one host. Certainly isopropyl alcohol and aflatoxin B seem to be found in large quantities if a parasite is present and this creates a carcinogenic environment for the host.

Aflatoxin B seems to be produced by certain parasites and is highly toxic. Linus Pauling, the champion of vitamin C, claimed that large doses in excess of one gram of vitamin C a day would have a positive effect on some cancer sufferers. One possible explanation is that vitamin C has been found to neutralise aflatoxin B.

Yeasts

Another common phenomenon is yeast infection. Usually the result of taking too many antibiotics, it can have a similar effect on the host's body to parasite infection. When antibiotics are prescribed, they kill not only the offending bacterium of the illness, but also most of the 'good guys' inside the digestive system. This allows the yeast to grow and multiply. Rather like mushrooms, they have a matrix of fine roots, which go across the intestinal lining and into the blood supply. This means that certain things that shouldn't, pass almost unfiltered into the blood system with toxic results. It is estimated that up to 70 per cent of the UK population has an over-development of yeasts.

One effect of both parasites and yeasts is similar. They deplete the body of nourishment and vitamins, and especially B vitamins, whilst increasing the level of toxins in the host's body and weakening their immune system.

Viruses

Up to 20 per cent of people have some sort of long-term viral infection. The herpes virus is now being linked to some vaginal and prostate cancers. There are nine types of herpes virus, only one being passed sexually. Others include shingles, chicken pox and glandular fever. Indeed some cases of breast cancer appear to follow an attack of shingles. There is a link between human papilloma virus (HPV) and several cancers. Viruses are also linked to cancer of the liver and blood. Again viral infection robs the host of nourishment, increases levels of toxins and weakens the immune system, often in quite a localised area.

Bacteria
The relatively common bacterium helicobacter pylori, which only recently was linked to stomach ulcers, is now being associated with stomach cancer. It can be eliminated using a cocktail of antibiotics. Similar bacterial infections are also linked to bladder cancer.

Human Papilloma Virus (HPV)

HPV is the fastest spreading sexually transmitted disease. Usually the virus is simply cleared out of the body in a year or so, although in some cases it may remain dormant for a very long time. More than half of all sexually active Americans will carry the virus at some point in their lives. Men are unlikely to even know they have it.

HPV enters through tiny abrasions in the skin and condoms are not much use as mere skin contact is usually enough to pass on the virus. No reliable tests exist and there is currently no treatment or cure.

Worse it is a 'smart' virus and even the immune system does not seem to notice its presence because it multiplies prodigiously inside a skin cell, which then dies. These dead skin cells are literally virus 'pods' ready to spread to the next host.

HPV causes cervical cancer, cancers of the genitalia and anus and is implicated in several others.

To put figures on this about 500,000 women worldwide contract cervical cancer each year and only 50 per cent survive five years.

Vaccines are being developed, and one by Merck Sharpe and Dohme is in final trials now. It seems effective with two strains of HPV that account for 70 per cent of cervical cancers. However it is preventative and has no effect if the man or woman is already a carrier. Preventative vaccines also bring with them a debate over at what age people should be vaccinated, particularly as the age at which first sexual contact takes place is reducing.

Although the medical world says there is no way of detecting HPV presence, some homeopaths believe they can detect it, and this may be a route to explore if you are concerned. Indeed, some homeopaths also believe they can eradicate HPV from the body.

For the moment the best answer seems to be long-term monogamy!

The important point is that many seemingly normal people may well be carriers of parasites, yeasts or viruses and need to deal with them. It is possible to be tested for many viruses, plus parasites and yeast and bacteria, by doctors, homeopaths and specialist clinics.

Where cancer sufferers are concerned it is imperative that tests are carried out to see if they are infected, so that these 'enemies of the state' can be eradicated quickly if they are detected.

Many viruses can be treated using modern drugs. Parasites can be eradicated over time :

- By taking steps to cleanse your diet (eg using clean and filtered water, by removing uncooked meats and dairy products from your diet)
- By avoiding certain pollutants, eg isopropyl alcohol from personal products and pesticides
- By taking a number of natural products to remove the parasites or their toxic by-products, eg a mixture of natural ingredients like ground cloves, wormwood, garlic, ginger, anise and slippery elm with vitamin C (there are proprietary products you can buy).

Yeasts can be treated by using garlic, Pau d'Arco, caprylic acid and oregano. Again proprietary brands can be used. Yeast sufferers should also take acidophilus tablets in high strength form. (This is no bad thing for everybody. The stomach can lose its complete supply of good bacteria in just three days if you are unwell.)

In all three cases the immune system should be boosted with zinc 15 mgs, vitamin C 1gm slow release and B complex (especially biotin 0.3mgs).

Even if yeasts, parasites, and viruses do not actually cause cancer they do play their part in weakening the whole immune system by increasing toxins and removing vitamins. This makes the body much more vulnerable to contracting or sustaining cancer.

As an example of the influence of yeasts, Pau d'Arco for a long time was thought to have great anti-cancer benefits. But it is now thought that this is more likely to be due to the indirect effect of killing off yeasts rather than any direct effect on cancer cells.

(iv) A self-debilitating mental attitude

This is a huge subject and the reason why a whole section of this book (section III) is devoted to 'mind over matter'.

Often sufferers are not being true to themselves. They like to please others and put others first, often neglecting their own well-being. Because emotional factors like strong feelings of guilt or unworthiness, they seek peer group approval and put up with unhappy jobs or unhappy surroundings (including people who put them down). As a result they often live in environments that just don't 'fit', they are neglecting their own true happiness, they have little sense of purpose or emotional reward. They put up with undue stresses and problems because they feel it is their lot.

Their inability to be true to themselves is linked to a lowered self-esteem and self-worth. They do not take time for themselves and this leads to greater imbalances between the life they lead and the life they need, at emotional and physical levels. As section III will show, this directly leads to a reduced body energy level and a measurable decline in the immune system of up to 30 per cent.

Everybody should put themselves through an emotional and physical 'health check' regularly and ask what makes them happy, what makes them unhappy, what causes most stress. Defining a sense of purpose that would fulfil them, planning a lifestyle that provides time for mental and physical 'nourishment', relaxation and stimulation and removing the creators of toxins (including people) that influence their lives.

Depression has strong links to cancer. Depression lowers

oxygen levels in the blood and cells by up to 30 per cent (and thus cancer, which hates oxygen, can thrive).

Depression also affects the cellular environment negatively through the eicosanoid system (see Q19) and it is no wonder that depression alone has been linked to 30 to 40 per cent of all cancers. *Time* magazine in January 2003 carried a thorough review.

Q10. Which environmental carcinogens may cause cancer?

'It isn't pollution that's harming the environment. It's the impurities in our air and water that's doing it'. These words of wisdom were provided by none less a person than the former Vice-President of the USA, Dan Quayle.

As said before, the onset of cancerous cells is a multi-step process and that environmental, lifestyle and diet issues individually are usually not enough to cause cancer. A predisposition and infection are also co-factors. However, let's start with a look at some of the environmental factors that we come into contact with almost every day. I do not want to labour any of these points, just give you a brief picture.

(i) Water

'Even the Archbishop of Canterbury is 80 per cent water', said J B Haldane a notable biochemist more than half a century ago. Water is vital to all our bodily functions, the provision of fuels to our cells and the removal of waste and toxins. Athletes or people in extreme terrains who have a 10 per cent fall in their hydration level experience a 50 per cent fall in everything from their energy levels to their ability to concentrate.

Tap water, depending upon your location, can have a mixture of parasites, heavy and toxic metals like copper and lead from the pipes, pesticides, nitrites, and aluminium from the water purification process, oestrogen, and even radioactivity. In some places the level of chlorine at certain times of the day can exceed levels recommended for swimming pools. Chlorine can change the body's pH and kill the friendly bacteria essential for intestinal health.

Oestrogen is a particularly worrying component in recycled tap waters. Caused by the increased use of the birth control pill and HRT, some lakes and rivers have been shown to have a disproportionate number of female fish, with male fish losing their male characteristics. Certainly changing diets and factors such as oestrogen consumption have seen a change in the ratio of boys to girls born in the UK. A hundred years ago more boys were born, but now this has been reversed. There is also concern that oestrogen is a factor in causing human sperm counts to fall.

Boiling the water doesn't help much as this merely serves to concentrate some of the metals and pollutants. (You would need to distil the water rather than simply boil it, but nutrients would then be lost).

Bottled water also has its problems, as plastic bottles are known to leach out carcinogens (phthalates which are oestrogen mimics) into the water. Far safer is water in glass bottles.

Most water filters are quite good, but they are limited in their effectiveness. The only really safe solution is a serious reverse osmosis water filter, but even some of those can be ineffective with oestrogen, and the irony is the water produced is felt by some people to be too clean!

(ii) Silent killers?

Radiation

The Royal College of Radiologists believes that as many as 250 cases of fatal cancers are caused per year by X-rays. Professor Gofman of UCLA believes that as many as 75 per cent of breast cancers are actually caused by medical X-rays in the USA. X-rays during pregnancy have been directly linked to a 50 per cent increase in childhood leukaemia.

CAT scans give you a much higher dose of radiation than normal X-rays, whilst MRI scans subject the body to forces 50,000 times those normally encountered on earth. Research is currently underway to see if MRI scans actually cause cancer.

Mammograms are the subject of huge debate. They provide approximately 1,000 times the dose of an X-ray.

Dense breast tissue is risky breast tissue and is linked to breast cancer. Unfortunately Western women's high levels of oestrogen, coupled with diet and lifestyle, results in dense tissue. However, the denser the tissue the less likely a mammogram is to spot an early developing tumour. It is a serious conundrum facing doctors and all women in the West.

Radiation from medical treatments is also a concern. Interestingly, the health correspondent of *The Times* in November 2002, seeking to play down fears of the damage caused by a dirty terrorist bomb, which would scatter radiation dust in the air, claimed it was only similar to the dose from a whole body X-ray. If true this would make a mammogram as 'dirty' as 1,000 Al Qaeda bombs!

Electromagnetic fields (EMFs)
Every one of us has a natural body energy field around us and it can be dangerous and unhealthy to interfere with this. Dr Reiter of the University of Texas, San Antonio, leads a team of researchers who have linked EMFs to the suppression of melatonin production and to an increased cancer risk.

Nine studies in the UK show that relatively low levels of EMFs from power cables, pylons or mains electricity are directly linked to an increased risk of childhood cancer, especially leukaemia. This has been confirmed in the USA and Sweden.

What of sockets either side of the bed head, TVs in the bedroom or electric blankets? All can be unwanted sources of localised EMFs.

It would be wise to reduce your exposure to TV and VDU screens. TVs should be 3 metres away from the viewer as a minimum and covered from view in a bedroom at night, even if they are switched off. VDUs should always be switched off when not in use and less powerful alternatives, for example, powerbooks, used where possible.

And it is possible to live on dangerous fault lines of electromagnetic energy. Transmitters on hills can have magnetic fields lying between them, causing hot spots.

In January 2002 the small Spanish village of Valladolid won a landmark victory to remove 36 mobile phone transmitters installed on a building 50 metres from the local primary school.

In the 18 months since the masts had been erected four of the children had developed cancer, yet prior to it there had not been a case for 34 years.

Other houses have quite unexplained magnetic fields running

through them, which appear not to be linked to power lines or to have geological sources. Dr Clarke of the UK Radiological Protection Board was quoted as saying: '*It could be the way the homes were wired or something about their supply, or their use of appliances.*'

Mobile phones

If you turn a phone on and it is making a call, when you place it next to a bucket of water 90 per cent of the phones ionising radiation will pass into the bucket of water. This phenomenon is called induction. In fact, only a small proportion of the power of a mobile phone is actually used in transmitting the call to the receiver mast; the rest goes into any nearby object, your head, your hand, your hips.

Dr Lennart Hardel has released two papers (the last in October 2002 – *International Journal of Radiation Biology*), linking mobile phones with malignant brain tumours.

The Finnish Radiation and Nuclear Safety Authority has reported its view that mobile phones caused activity in the cells lining the blood-brain barrier changing its ability to protect the brain from harmful substances.

Colorado University researchers have shown that frequent mobile phone users had significantly depressed melatonin levels (see Q18).

A Swedish study involving 2,900 people concluded that people who hold their phones to their heads more than double their risks of a tumour, which typically takes three to four years to develop.

The Environmental Health Trust concludes, '*20–80 per cent of the electromagnetic radiation generated by mobile phones (depending upon the make) is directly absorbed into the user's brain.*' And, '*A few minutes exposure to cell-phone type radiation can transform a 5 per cent active cancer into a 95 per cent active cancer*'.

Around 25 per cent of mobile phones are used by the under 18s, and according to a report in *The Ecologist*, children are most in danger because their skulls are thinner, allowing the radiation to penetrate further into their brains. With a developing nervous system they are more prone to memory impairment and immune deficiency. A recent Spanish research study confirms this. A child using a mobile phone, even for a very short period, experiences a significant slowing of brain function for up to 50 minutes.

Roger Coghill, an anti-mobile phone biologist has recently been defeated in his case to have warning labels introduced. But he is quite clear, *'Anyone who uses a mobile phone for longer than 20 minutes quite literally should have their head examined'*.

Radon

Radon is a radioactive gas formed by the natural radioactive decay of uranium in rock, soil and water. Low levels of uranium occur widely in the earth's crust and some areas have more than others.

Radon itself is colourless, tasteless, odourless and chemically inert. Unless you test for it, you'd never know it was there. Once produced by the uranium, it bubbles up through the ground into the air above.

The problem comes if you are in a higher-than-average radon area. Radon accumulates inside homes, building up to high levels that are not easily dispersed. Electrically charged atoms from the radon attach themselves to dust particles, which can be inhaled. Inside your lungs the decaying particles produce radiation, which has the potential to damage lung tissue.

The Surgeon General in the USA has warned that radon is the second leading cause of lung cancer and is a 'serious public health problem'. (*National Academy of Sciences*). It is estimated that 40,000 cases of lung cancer are caused each year in the USA by radon. Problem areas in the UK include Wales and the South West, but there are pockets in the Midlands, north of Manchester and north east of Edinburgh.

There is also evidence of a synergistic effect between radon and smoking, which increases risk by 55 per cent, (*National Safety Council, Washington*).

If you are worried about radon or lung cancer, you can get your home checked. (Details in appendix II.)

Gas appliances

Although there is absolutely no evidence to link gas appliances to cancer, there is concern that exhaust products from them weaken the immune system and have been linked, for example, to arthritis. Levels of nitrogen dioxide in homes with gas boilers and gas cookers may exceed government levels laid down as constituting severe pollution in city environments.

Diesel fumes
Diesel fumes cause similar problems to radon. The fumes are particulate, and the 'nasties' can be inhaled into the deepest corners of your lungs. US research is quite clear about the links to lung cancer.

(iii) Medicines, antibiotics, anti-inflammatories and vaccines

In their book *Brain Fitness*, Dr Robert Goldman and Dr Ronald Klatz, the President of the American Academy of Anti-Ageing Medicine, define both antibiotics and anti-inflammatories as 'brain poisons'. They have been shown to have links with cancer. It is better to take aspirin, which seems to be gaining a reputation as an anti-cancer agent because of its anti-inflammatory powers. (See Q20.)

A leading US authority (Moore) claimed that prescription drugs pose the largest group of avoidable toxins available to Americans. Another survey of 240 high usage US prescription drugs stated that over half contained known carcinogens and posed serious risk of cancer at normal dosage levels. Many drugs have not been around long enough for us to know what their long-term effect as carcinogens is likely to be.

Why not go to a cranial osteopath, homeopath or acupuncturist next time you are ill? No one ever said these people could cause cancer and they may well find an underlying reason for the problem, a solution which may not require antibiotics or drugs in the long term.

Vaccinations are a cause for some concern, particularly as there have been no in-depth studies on their safety in relation to cancer. The arguments are based on the toxic way the vaccines are prepared, the impurities contained such as mercury, and the chance of the viruses used in the vaccines themselves causing cancer.

Even the vitamin industry is not immune to selling us carcinogens. Some multivitamins and minerals in pill form can contain toxic heavy metals, whilst some mass produced fish oils, especially from fish caught in coastal waters, can contain dioxins.

(iv) Over exposure to sunlight

Strong sunlight seems able to provide all the multi-step processes in cancer formation and well documented evidence links this to skin cancer, particularly in people who take white bodies for a two-week trip to the sun. Unfortunately, sunscreens may not give us the protection we had hoped; some have recently been banned in Scandanavian countries for containing carcinogenic ingredients. (Look for PABA free products). You should avoid overexposure especially at the start of a trip, particularly lying in the sun in hot countries between 11am and 3pm.

People should be wary of sunbeds too. Professor Andrew Tannahill, chief executive officer of the Health Education Board for Scotland says, *'Weekly use exposes people to six times the annual dose of UV radiation. Sunbeds have always been suspected of causing skin cancer. The evidence is now clear.'*

(v) Insecticides and pesticides

Pesticides have been implicated in many illnesses ranging from birth defects to cancer. The link between cancer and pesticide exposure is well documented. Pesticides used at home, for example, to kill flies, on dog collars and to eradicate garden insects, links to a four-fold increase in childhood leukaemia and a greater incidence of brain tumours. Children under 14 whose gardens are sprayed with herbicides have a four times greater incidence of connective tissue tumours.

Some commercial apple trees are sprayed 10–12 times. After picking, apples are waxed so that they look good in shops. It is then virtually impossible to wash the residue of the pesticides off the apple skin. Broccoli, a wonderful source of vitamins C and E, collects pesticide under the florets making washing it out equally difficult. Organic is the only safe option, although even then you must be certain of the origin.

The US Natural Resources Defence Council in their 1989

report concluded that eight pesticides in particular, commonly used on fruit and vegetables, and regularly consumed by pre-school children, made them more likely to develop cancer later in life.

There are believed to be high residues of many carcinogens in fruits, grains and vegetables, yet there is little legislation, and health warnings are not apparent.

Only recently the US Environmental Protection Agency's estimate of the amount of such residues you can safely consume in a lifetime was shown to be exceeded by a baby's total consumption in its first year of life.

This is made more acute by the finding that the young have a much higher susceptibility to carcinogens than their parents do. Tests on young mice show as much as 100 per cent mortality with carcinogens that have no effect on the parents. There are also very real concerns about the consumption of carcinogens by pregnant women and the long-term effects on the unborn child.

(vi) Air quality

Oxygen is the enemy of cancer. At school we learned that air is 21 per cent oxygen. Several hundred thousand years ago this figure was over 30 per cent. In polluted cities it can be as low as 12 per cent and life ceases below 7 per cent.

To beat cancer you need clean efficient lungs taking in clean, oxygenated air. Most of us compound the problem of poor air quality because we simply do not breathe properly, taking short, almost superficial breaths from chest movements rather than deep breaths using our diaphragms. As a result, stagnant air collects in the lower third to half of our lungs leaving them full of toxins that need to be expelled to avoid our systems being polluted. The action of yawning is caused by this stagnation and the polluted body feeling tired and listless. External pollutants like carbon monoxide from exhausts and cigarettes makes matters worse; not only does it take up space in your lungs but it binds with the haemoglobin, reducing its ability to carry oxygen to the cells.

Everybody, as a minimum, needs to spend time going for energetic walks in the countryside, avoiding polluted places and taking time to breathe fresh air deeply. Early morning light exercise, ideally in fresh air and using deep breaths, does you good. It is interesting that an important part of the Chinese approach to cancer therapy involves deep breathing exercises.

(vii) Toxins in household products, toiletries, and cosmetics

Carcinogens surround us and are contained in everything from toothpaste to shampoos, and household cleaners to mouthwashes. Most plastic packaging contains carcinogens that leach out into the food and liquid.

In 1995 David Steinman and Samuel Epstein co-wrote *The Safe Shoppers Bible*. This book is awesome in its review of 4,000 US consumer products including household products, cosmetic, toiletries, and food detailing lists of carcinogenic ingredients.

Epstein is also chairman of the Cancer Prevention Coalition in the USA and worked with Ralph Nader to name and shame the 'Dirty Dozen' consumer products. In 1995 he named toxic ingredients in a number of products including some household cleaners, talcum powder (directly linked to ovarian cancer), permanent hair colour, make-up, a weed killer, toothpaste, and a hair conditioner. In 2001 he wrote a book entitled *Unreasonable Risk*, listing two pages of carcinogens found in US cosmetic and personal care products, of which 40 actually feature on labels (open ingredients) whilst 30 are hidden. Even in the open category, seven are proven 'genotoxins' ie in animal or human studies they have been shown to induce genetic damage and the mainstream petrochemical industry admits there is no way of determining thresholds or safety levels. Over the last five years just a few of his concerns have been:

- A wide range of ingredients in **shampoos** break down to form formaldehyde. Polysorbates may be contaminated with 1, 4-dioxane which is carcinogenic.
- **Lipsticks** contain BHA, sodium, saccharin and artificial colourings all possible carcinogens.
- Possible carcinogens cited in **toothpastes** include saccharin, and sodium lauryl sulphate (SLS) which is also found in **mouthwashes** and **soaps**. SLS is known as a skin irritant. It can

damage the immune system and, as a mutagen, harm the cells' genetic make-up.

- Any **hair dye** containing a phenylenediamine-based ingredient may induce human cancer. The EU is currently looking at links between dark hair dyes and the incidence of bladder cancer.
- Ethoxylated alcohols, most often found in **liquid detergents** and **soaps** (including many 'natural' brands), can contain 1,4-dioxane.
- Aluminium in **antiperspirants** is linked to increased risk of Alzheimer's. Antiperspirants may also contain another 10 ingredients, 'wholly unnecessary for the product's effectiveness' and listed under the heading of carcinogens.

The list seems endless. Every free-thinking person should buy the book and look for non-toxic alternative products.

Two of his prime concerns are that there is no proper regulation of what goes into many of the products you buy for your home and that, even if an ingredient is disclosed on the label, the great majority of people have no idea of its toxicity.

He is also worried about the mix of chemicals you come into contact with everyday. For example, using two different products on the human face may cause a chemical reaction between some of their ingredients, which subsequently produces a carcinogen. The skin is a known carrier, rather than a barrier, for many ingredients and toxins. Twenty-four hour exposure to SLS, one of the wetting agents used in many skin care products, has been shown to damage the protein layer of the skin making it more porous.

In case you don't feel that making the skin on your hands more porous is much of a problem, consider this: a recent study showed that the new Euro coin when taped to the back of the hands of members of a research group, resulted in severe irritation and even blistering after 48 hours.

Clearly members of the general public are not going to go around like this in their normal daily lives, but the problem was put down to nickel in the coins. Nickel is believed to be linked to prostate cancer as it can substituted for zinc in the prostate. Making your skin more porous is not a good idea.

It has been calculated that American men use on average 10

personal care products per day whilst women use 13 personal care and six cosmetic products. Some products like hand soaps are used more than once. This makes the number of possible carcinogenic 'hits' on your body very high, even for babies and young children.

Recent studies have shown that American women can have almost four times the level of toxins in their bloodstreams that American men have, and it has been concluded that this is largely due to their greater usage of cosmetics, toiletries and household products.

Q11. What are the main lifestyle factors that increase my risk of cancer?

(i) Alcohol

Alcohol is a chemical poison and has many negative effects, but particularly it overworks the liver potentially causing damage, produces dangerous free radicals, and causes immune system depletion. It is also a neurotoxin damaging the brain and the nervous system. In November 2002, a study linked alcohol consumption with breast cancer in women. Apparently it is thought to stimulate oestrogen production, and a woman's risk of breast cancer increases by 6 per cent for every drink consumed per day (*British Journal of Cancer* vol 87). Alcohol is also implicated in oesophagal, stomach and colon cancer. An occasional glass of Cabernet Sauvignon may have antioxidant benefits. Better to stick to red grape juice. People with cancer should avoid alcohol because it puts stress on an already overworked liver.

(ii) Tobacco

The packets have health warnings. They are there for a reason. Smoking causes severe free radical release in the body. It is madness to smoke without accepting you are greatly increasing your odds of getting cancer especially after 55 years of age. If you smoke, stop now!

Statistically, even one cigarette a day has the same odds of causing cancer as 20.

Worryingly even non-smokers get smoke-related lung cancer. Cancer Research UK announced findings in autumn 2002 that showed people living with a 20 a day smoker were exposed to six-times the smoke levels of people living in a smoke-free household.

People who work in smoky environments are at risk. Roy Castle's death was attributed to passive smoking; although a non-smoker himself he frequently entertained and played the trumpet in smoke-filled clubs.

The Government should ban smoking in all public places; it is a nonsense to subject children and non-smokers to the selfish whim of a minority of the population.

Women are especially at risk from tobacco smoke. Women have two X-chromosomes in their DNA, men only have one in their DNA. A gene on that X-chromosome causes a carcinogenic factor to appear in the airways of smokers. So women smokers have roughly twice the risk of men who smoke the same number of cigarettes. (Siegfried, University of Pittsburgh). Oestrogen further increases the presence of this factor. Your daughter must not smoke. If they smoke, girls in their sexually formative years, especially those taking the pill as well, increase their risk of breast cancer by a staggering 70 per cent later in life.

(iii) The Pill and HRT

An excess of oestrogen, besides depleting vitamin B, has been shown to have specific links to breast and prostate cancer. Oestrogen binds with receptors on the cell's surface inducing it to turn rogue.

Even in small amounts, it is a very powerful immunosuppressant. In excessive amounts, oestrogen is a very powerful and very dangerous hormone in women.

Two hundred or more years ago women naturally regulated their oestrogen levels. Their periods started around the age of 16 to 18 and ended age 38 to 40; they had four babies on average and breast-fed them for nine months to two years. Nowadays, changing diets and lifestyles, less babies and breast-feeding has increased the average number of periods a woman has by about 60 per cent or so. Thus the exposure to these oestrogen peaks has also grown significantly.

A Swedish study has linked both late menopause and short menstrual cycles with increased rates of lung cancer.

But it is breast cancer that produces the greatest alarm. The World Health Organisation (WHO) in 1985 linked the oestrogen contraceptive pill to increases in invasive cancers. Nowhere more so than in breast cancer.

To have ever taken the pill increases a woman's chance of breast cancer by 26 per cent; to take it into her 30's increases risk by 58 per cent and in her 40's by 144 per cent. (Cancer Research UK).

HRT creates the same sort of problems. A recent report in the *Lancet* (Vol 360, pages 942-4) concluded that there is a significant increase in the risk of breast cancer, strokes and blood clots on the lungs. HRT was determined to be the actual cause of some breast cancers in women taking it. A 2002 US study on HRT was stopped because of cancer and heart problems, and figures indicated an increased cancer risk at over 27 per cent. Cancer Research UK was adamant in a press release in October 2002 that the risks of HRT outweighed the protective benefits. (Progesterone does not cause the same problems, and there is even some indication that it reduces the risks of ovarian cancer by 50 per cent according to Dr Schildkraut at The Duke Cancer Centre, Carolina.)

(iv) A sedentary lifestyle and being overweight

We have already talked about the need to have movement to get the lymph system flowing and reduce pollution around the cells.

We also covered the reasons why overweight people are 40 per cent more likely than the norm to develop a cancer.

But how do you know if you are in the danger zone?

Most measurements seem too complicated for the normal person. I'm a fully qualified fitness trainer and the Body Mass Index (BMI), which is the official system we are taught to use, is totally meaningless to the average person. It might be helpful to know your fat content and there are simple machines, probably at your local gym, that will tell you. Weight to height is not always strictly relevant because a body builder who puts on muscle may find he weighs more than a slightly fat friend of the same height, simply because muscle weighs more than fat. Bone density also plays a part.

However the following charts give you some clue as to whether or not you are at risk.

MEN				
Height	Underweight	Healthy Weight	Overweight	Obese
5 ft 1in	below 48	48 -63	63-74	74+
5 ft 4in	below 53	53-68	68-80	80+
5 ft 7in	below 59	59-73	73-86	86+
5 ft 10in	below 64	64-79	79-93	93+
6 ft 1in	below 69	69-85	85-103	103+
All weights shown are in kilograms				

WOMEN				
Height	Underweight	Healthy Weight	Overweight	Obese
5ft 0in	below 44	44-56	56-67	67+
5ft 3in	below 48	48-60	60-72	72+
5ft 6in	below 53	53-66	66-78	78+
5ft 9in	below 57	57-72	72-85	85+
6ft 0in	below 62	62-79	79-93	93+
All weights shown are in kilograms				

I really must caution that these figures are just generally indicative and more individually accurate figures can be made from an estimation of your fat content linked to height and bone structure.

(v) My mother's pregnancy!

There are some dangers you can do little about!

Scientists have analysed 10,000 cases of children's cancer using the British National Registry of Childhood Tumours, and concluded your **mother's age** during her pregnancy makes a lot of difference.

Children with acute lymphoblastic leukaemia, which accounts

for a quarter of all childhood cancers were born more often to older mothers.

Mothers aged between 35 and 39 were 30 per cent more likely, and mothers aged 40 and above were 88 per cent more likely than those of 25 to 29 to have a child with this disease.

Unconnected to this, Swedish researchers have shown that three-quarters of 34 **perfumes and perfume toiletry products** tested, contain phthalates (oestrogen mimics) and particularly di-ethylhexyl phthalate. The urine of American women, in a second study, showed the by-products, and at levels many times higher than in corresponding men.

Numerous studies have shown that these phthalates are linked to male reproductive problems in boys born to these women; undescended testicles and testicular cancer being two of them.

Your cancer could have started before you were born.

(vi) Stresses and lifestyle

This area is complex and is tackled in far more detail in section III of this book. For now, here are three examples of the problems that can be caused:

- Stress particularly depletes B vitamins and causes the production of steroids in the body. This has a negative effect on the immune system, the endocrine system and localised cellular biochemistry. All these lead to an increased risk of rogue cell production and a failure by the immune system to cope.
- There has been a study undertaken by SAS (the airline) linking irregular sleeping patterns in long haul stewardesses with depleted levels of melatonin and increased risks of cancer.
- Depression causes physiological changes in the blood count and reduces the blood's oxygen carrying ability. Since cancer cells hate oxygen, depression actually favours cancer. Depression also brings about localised hormonal changes and localised toxin production both of which increase the risk of forming cancer cells.

You need to spend time on your body and your mind.

Q12. What are the main dietary factors that increase my risk of cancer?

The types of cancer that are most affected (positively and negatively) by diet are those which are largely hormone driven (eg oesophageal, liver, pancreatic, colon, breast, prostate, stomach). Throughout this book there are frequent mentions of diet so I will not labour the point. The essential discipline is, 'Eat less meat, less animal fat and more vegetables and fruit. Think nourishment; think nutritious.'

(i) Dairy foods

We are the only animals that drink the milk of different species such as cows, goats and sheep. Normal milk contains extra hormones that you don't want like oestrogen, factors that affect your insulin levels, pesticide residues from fields, animal fat and so on. If the cows have been fed growth hormones and anti-biotics, traces of those will be found in their milk too.

Professor Jane Plant, who herself had breast cancer, has looked into the effect of dairy products on breast and prostate cancers concluding that there is a direct link. She believes it is an, 'all or none' situation. Even taking in small amounts of dairy (for example, a bar of chocolate, milk in a coffee, even a 'live organic yoghurt') increases the risk of these two cancers. Like smoking, you can't be a non-smoker who still just has one a day.

Scandanavian research in 2000 concluded that 'there is a direct link between consumption of dairy foods and testicular and prostrate cancer rates'.

Part of the problem concerns Insulin Growth Factor (IGF1) which can throw normal hormone levels out and affect cellular environments negatively whilst increasing oestrogen levels. IGF1 has been shown to pass from the intestines into the bloodstream in mice in small amounts (6 per cent) but this increases to 68 per cent if cassein is present. Cassein is a milk protein.

In another test, even a small amount of butter, or margarine (which often contains dairy products), was found to suppress the body's detoxification enzymes just when you need them (Strang Cancer Prevention Centre, New York).

(ii) Meat, animal fat and farmed fish

Animal fat is a saturated fat. It promotes all manner of cancers and animal fat should be cut to a minimum. It stimulates prostaglandins (see eicosanoids later) in the body which act as inflammatory agents and demand attention from your immune system, thus weakening it. If all this weren't bad enough, meat contains large volumes of the animal's own hormones (which you can reduce by cooking well) and often antibiotics and hormones given to the animal to make it grow bigger and stronger. Farmed fish is not much better, often containing growth hormones, antibiotics and even colourants, like the false pink of smoked salmon. Farmed salmon contains 20 per cent more fat than its wild predecessor.

(iii) Fats and oils in general

By and large fats and oils are bad for you, whatever their source. Any and all fats (even good oils like olive oil) drive up oestrogen levels in the body and increase the risk of hormone based cancers like breast and prostate cancers. Fats also impair the function of white blood cells and thus your immune system. Vegetarians do twice as well as meat eaters in the ability of their immune system to seek and destroy rogue cells. Reducing consumption of fats and oils makes an enormous difference, although of course you must not cut them out completely as they are essential to the normal functioning of the body.

Fats and oils can be classified under three headings:

- **Saturated fats.** These are the worst for you. As with smoking, the end product of eating animal fat or a hydrogenated vegetable oil is a free radical that will cause premature ageing and potentially cancer. This is why you should limit your consumption of red meats and all fried snack foods like crisps, onion rings, peanuts and fast foods, which are invariably covered in this 'killer' fat.

- **Polyunsaturated fats and oils.** A while back these were thought to be the breakthrough and a generation of sunflower oils and margarines purporting to be healthy was launched. They are far better for you than saturated fats and the list includes safflower, sunflower, soybean oil and peanut oil, but they are now believed to be less good for you that was originally claimed.

- **Monounsaturated fats and oils.** Found, for example, in olive oil, walnut oil, flaxseed oil and macadamia nut oil. But beware of some margarines which you think are 100 per cent olive oil. They can contain other fats, oils and even dairy products.

It must be remembered that consuming large amounts of carbohydrate, in excess of your needs, results in increasing your fat stores. Indeed, the Harvard Medical School has just published a rethink of the high carbohydrate, low fat 'idealised' diet decreed by governments 20 years ago. Low carbohydrates, low animal fats, good levels of fruit and vegetables and oils from nuts and seeds and oily fish are some of its features.

(iv) Refined foods and processed foods

White flour is refined and has had a lot of the goodness removed. Look for wholemeal or wholegrain. Don't be misled by brown breads that claim to be 'wheat grain' or 'malted', which is merely refined white flour with added colouring. In malt bread, for example, the malt has dyed the refined white bread brown.

All processed foods suffer in the processing. TV dinners and ready-made meals are packages of danger. These foods have to have preservatives to enhance their shelf life, and many are a blend of ingredients and chemicals to achieve an acceptable taste.

Recent studies in Scandinavia have shown that processed foods such as biscuits, breakfast cereals, crispbreads, crisps and especially overcooked chips contain acrylamides. These are produced when the cooking process exceeds 120°C. Acrylamides are highly toxic.

Many healthy fruit juices are really processed sources of sugar. A famous 'healthy' American natural grape juice declared on the bottle that it contained no vitamin C but it clearly had high levels of sugars. Processing destroys nourishment.

(v) Preservatives

Dried meats, pepperoni, hams, sausages and other processed

meats usually contain highly toxic nitrites. One study in America directly linked hot dog consumption to cancer in children. E numbers are another area for concern and pickling with vinegar is linked to stomach and throat cancers. Smoked meats and fish are not much better.

(vi) Salt, sugar

Both refined salt and sugar negatively affect your endocrine system. It is estimated we eat 10 times too much salt per day on average but beware, because most salt and sugar is hidden. Breakfast cereals, a loaf of bread, chicken nuggets and hundreds of processed foods manipulate the salt and sugar content to achieve a more popular taste. Fizzy soft drinks can have 10 spoonfuls of sugar per can.

(vii) Caffeine

Caffeine is a poison and is found in soft drinks, coffee, tea and chocolate. It depletes the body of vitamins, especially B vitamins, which are required for healthy cell maintenance and division. It also has a negative effect on the immune system.

(viii) Aspartame?

According to the UK Brain Tumour Foundation, an increase in brain tumours has been noted since aspartame was introduced into the food market in 1981. There is a school of thought, that Aspartame, which is found in a wide variety of diet drinks and yoghurts as the low calorie sweetener, is a neurotoxin and carcinogen. In laboratory tests it has been shown to cause aggressive brain tumours in rats. The arguments continue. Clinical tests are being conducted in the UK specifically looking at links between aspartame and child brain tumours at the moment. Meanwhile there is absolutely no evidence for these claims or rumours where humans are concerned.

(ix) Saccharin

There are a number of US studies with both animals and humans linking saccharin and bladder cancer.

(x) Poor diet and poor eating habits

Eating too few vegetables, insufficient fruit, no fibre, too much animal fat, burnt food, fried food, too many chips and crisps, too much sugar and salt, microwaved food; question 21 covers this in far more detail.

———————

There are many other possible carcinogens around but as I said at the beginning, this is about reducing the odds. Not smoking, limiting alcohol intake, avoiding fried foods, fats and red meats, dairy and caffeine, the pill, limiting exposure to extreme sunshine and clearing toxic products out of your house would be good and simple places to start and they will give you better odds for avoiding cancer. If you have cancer then they are actions you are strongly and urgently advised to consider.

Q13. What exactly is the immune system?

We have several defence systems in the body which protect us from outside attack. The main one of these is the immune system. A foreign body such as a virus or bacterium entering your body is called an antigen. Viruses and bacteria come in all shapes and sizes and have a complicated coat of protein and fats. Think of them as being like the hundreds of different shaped pieces of a jigsaw puzzle. Each invader of a different illness (eg measles or meningitis) has its own specific shape format.

The first thing that happens is that one or two of these invading pieces of jigsaw puzzle is carted off to the 'police station', the local lymph node (for example in your armpits). After a couple of days certain of your white blood cells (called B-lymphocytes) have measured up the invading jigsaw exactly and produced a protein coat (or antibody), which can exactly envelop and neutralise it.

Meanwhile the other identical invaders have been multiplying rapidly. The body now makes lots of tailored coats or antibodies to neutralise these. This can take a lot of effort and biochemical reaction, which is why you often have a fever. The masses of neutralised and now harmless cells are then removed by the 'clean up squad' called phagocytes and the liver and kidneys work overtime to break all these dead cells up and clear them from the body via the intestines.

However the B-lymphocytes have to be careful not to start neutralising your own good cells. Your thymus gland produces T-lymphocytes, a pair of which actually tell the B-lymphocytes what to do. They are sort of recognition agents monitoring all things as they pass by in the bloodstream. (As we will see later both melatonin and beta-carotene build T cell volume in the thymus). They sort out rogue invaders from normal good cells and sound the alert. There are many different formats for T cells and they are very clever search agents.

But T cells also work outside the blood stream at the cellular level too. Here they help reject large bacteria, yeasts, outside tissue transplants and cancerous cells. T cells take quite a while to do their monitoring and rejection job at the cellular level but they are crucial to fighting infection and cancers.

As one example, take the case of a man who had a kidney transplant. He was given immune system supressing drugs to stop rejection of the new transplanted tissue. A while later a routine body X-ray showed he was developing lung cancer, and it was discovered that the transplanted kidney had a very small cancer in it (the lung cancer was thus a secondary). The infected kidney was removed and the T cells got back to work and neutralised and cleared the lung cancer.

Healthy membranes of B-lymphocytes and T-lymphocytes are crucial to help the locking-on process, fitting the tailored coat over the rogue invader jigsaw piece.

These membranes contain fats which can be oxidised (literally, turned rancid) by free radicals. As we will see later, antioxidants (especially vitamin E) guard them and prevent this from happening.

Thus, a healthy thymus and clean and efficient liver and kidneys are all crucial to a good immune system.

The 'catch' is that with some cancers the immune system finds it very hard to distinguish between the cancerous cell and the normal one and this is why immunotherapy, which involves using interleukin to directly boost immune cells has had poor results in the past. The immune system is a very complex protector with a host of co-factors and helpers operating to make it work to its maximum.

Many cancers can be seen as a situation where the immune system, rather than identifying and kicking out the rogue cancer cell, merely tolerates its existence. In this case work has to be done to refocus and stimulate the immune system to get it back into full action. Sometimes the necessary kick can be provided by high dose vitamins, sometimes by reinvigorating the body energy systems, sometimes by drugs.

However, there is a chance with any cancer that a small percentage of up to 10 per cent, can successfully hide from the immune system. Genome work has identified two bits of your DNA string called BRCA1 and BRCA2. Originally these were incorrectly identified as breast cancer 'genes'. Actually they can be responsible for some prostate, colon, lung cancers and, maybe, many more types. These 'genes' are inherited and basically have the potential to switch off the immune system's identifying capabilities. If you are tested and have a high risk of these 'genes' you need to be extremely careful in your diet, lifestyle and environment so that you do not originate rogue cells in the first place, whilst trying to keep your immune system in tip-top condition. As I said, at the very most only 10 per cent of people have this problem.

Q14. What has my liver got to do with it?

All cancer patients suffer from liver inefficiency and overload. It can be overwhelmed by converting the lactic acid produced by cancer cells into glucose, by processing the by-products of neutralised dead cells, or by the negative effects of radiotherapy and chemotherapy on the body.

The liver contains a large number of bile ducts which, amongst other things, remove toxins from the blood and lymph systems and take them to the colon or intestines. There may well be stones, not a few but literally hundreds, clogging up these bile ducts. One estimate quoted that virtually every cancer patient suffered from gallstone blockage in the liver to some degree. Gallstones are caused by cholesterol deposits collecting around clumps of bacteria or pieces of dead parasite and it is not uncommon for cancer patients to have especially 'fatty' livers.

Far worse, the state of the liver can be severely worsened by parasites and by alcohol. As I said before, parasites can take any form, from microscopic ones, to a wide variety of flukes, which particularly inhabit the liver. Cancer patients must not drink alcohol under any circumstances; their liver has enough to do already.

All cancer patients, and people who want to be cancer free, should detox regularly and avoid the consumption of fats during that period. Proprietary detoxes can be purchased in health food stores and benefit the liver, bloodstream and whole body whilst parasite killers can be obtained from good vitamin suppliers. Natural sources of fibre like linseeds and psyllium can be eaten daily, and will also clean your colon as will aloe vera in tablets or liquid form. A clean colon helps you have a cleaner liver.

Choline, inositol, biotin, tumeric, methionine, and milk-thistle (*Selybum marianum*) all help to 'de-fat' and detox the liver. Herbs are also helpful. Artichoke helps the digestive process and fat breakdown and dandelion helps in fluid absorption.

But to clean it out and de-stone it takes serious effort. There is a detox involving Epsom salts, olive oil, and fresh pink grapefruit that seems to work but lays you low for a couple of days! (Epsom salts is an old-fashioned stomach cleaner and works very rapidly – see Appendix IV for details.)

When detoxing the body or the liver it is worth taking ornithine before going to sleep as the detoxification often results in poor sleep patterns.

Q15. How can I strengthen my immune system?

Firstly, a word about the use of supplements in general.

There is a school of thought that says, 'if we all ate properly we wouldn't need supplements'. This, quite simply, is not true.

For example, even if we ate properly we would be very unlikely to get more than 60 IU (International Units) of vitamin E inside us per day whereas 400 IU is a good level for cancer prevention. This is because our soil, and therefore the vegetables grown in it, have been depleted of nutrients over the last 100 years.

With anyone over the age of 65 we would expect lowered levels of coenzyme Q10 and melatonin both significant anti-cancer agents whose production in our bodies declines with age.

Even if you did regiment yourself to the ideal diet could you guarantee to eat it every day in the modern world? Could you get enough omega 3 if you went on a skiing trip, without taking cod liver oil pills, or get enough beta-carotene if you are on a two-day business trip?

Who says we are likely to eat properly anyway? The fact is that at least two thirds of the population do not. They like their waffles, crisps, croissants, butter, cheese, coffee, sugar, cakes and steaks. Half of their children never put a red, yellow or green vegetable in their mouths. Having such restricted diets risks people failing to ingest some of the more 'rare' trace elements such as boron, found to be vital in the anti-ageing process.

Virtually all the top anti-ageing experts in the USA take supplements.

And consider this; the US Senate concluded (and it is in the records) that laboratory tests prove that US farm soils are depleted as are the fruit, vegetables, nuts, eggs and even milk produced. It also concluded that people were developing mineral deficiencies and this could only be corrected by supplementation. And that was in the Senate minutes in 1936!

You can think of supplements in three ways:

- Insurance: for instance, a quality multivitamin and multi-mineral supplement ensures you ingest the trace elements you need every day
- Top up: for instance, vitamin C is water soluble, as is beta-carotene. They leave the body inside three hours. Supple-men-tation, especially using time-release pills, keeps a presence. Athletes lose a lot of vitamins during exercise especially vitamin B. No one eats enough vitamin E.
- Corrective: for instance, cod liver oil and coenzyme Q10 correct deficiencies in our food patterns, or those arising with age.

Supplements perform a highly useful role within a healthy diet especially when we need to kick-start a health programme. However it musts be recognised that they are supposed to 'supplement' and in the longer terms you should be restructuring your diet to reduce the dependency upon them as prime sources of vitamins. When you eat a red pepper or a carrot you get so much more than beta-carotene. Apart from other vitamins like vitamin C you get a wealth of supportive carotenoids, cofactors, and bioflavonoids, which are simply not present in a standard vitamin pill.

If you are unsure of what supplements you might need you can be tested for vitamin and mineral deficiency.

(i) Vitamin and other supplements

The next four questions and answers specifically address the whole issue of particular supplements, proven scientifically to have a positive effect in the fight against cancer. These sections include information on antioxidants (especially the 'magnificent six' – beta-carotene, vitamin C, vitamin E, selenium, zinc and coenzyme Q 10), vitamins and minerals, herbs and hormones.

(ii) Detoxing

These are ideas to strengthen your immune system:
- Cut out fats, animal fats, dairy and oils from your diet completely for a week or so.
- Take 200 mgs per day of milk-thistle (*Silybum marianum*), to

strengthen the liver. It helps it to detoxify itself and actively repairs liver damage.

- Liquid detoxes are simple to buy and use. There are also proprietary herbal detox mixtures available for liver cleansing including lipase, methionine, choline and inositol to help 'de-fat' the liver, plus biotin to help vitamin C work. Other herbal mixtures will help kidney function. The cleaning of the liver and kidneys for three to 10 days is essential after radiotherapy, chemotherapy or for the killing of yeast and parasites. The liver must be restored to full working order.
- Make your own juices and go on a juice diet; natural, freshly prepared juices have a serious fan club. There are plenty of books on the subject (see later).
- Drink copious amounts of water; at least 1.5 litres per day (and up to 3 litres during radiotherapy) this helps expel toxins and relieve the immune system.
- Take adequate fibre; this helps by expelling toxins from the colon after they have passed from the liver. Proprietary fibre brands containing psyllium, pectin (apple fibre), prune powder, flaxseed, Slippery Elm and hosts of other ingredients are easy to buy but must be taken with lots of water. Two tablespoons of linseeds sprinkled on the breakfast cereal are a simple to use source of fibre and omega 3.
- Have vegetarian days; and at least once per day, eat organic complete brown rice and eat two portions of fruit and six to eight of vegetables especially pulses such as lentils and mung beans.

(iii) Yoga, acupuncture, cranial osteopathy and reiki

Acupuncture will balance the body energy systems and natural pulses. It is very powerful and now recognised by the NHS. It works by linking the external aura or energy fields to the internal organs in a much more balanced and strengthening way. Like cranial osteopathy it helps get body energy where it is needed. Both of these, along with reiki have been proven to measurably increase the strength of the immune system.

Surprisingly (or not, depending upon your beliefs) certain forms of yoga, particularly Ashtanga, can strengthen your immune system by up to 30 per cent, again probably because they re-energise you, move your lymph system and they are known to expel toxins. New participants in these classes actually smell, as a huge volume of toxins is so quickly removed. All of these energy and immune boosters are covered in more detail later in the book.

Of course, the other way of strengthening your immune system is to cut out the carcinogen suspects listed in the previous answers. For example mobile phones in one study were claimed to reduce the localised immune system around the ear/head area by up to 30 per cent when held to the ear for a prolonged period.

This whole area is discussed more fully in section III.

Q16. What are the main antioxidants that could help?

In 1986, the US National Cancer Institute conducted a study in rural China amongst 30,000 people. Over a five year period the local population took the antioxidants beta-carotene, vitamin E and selenium. Within one to two years after commencing the study, cancer death rates started to fall, and after five years were 13 per cent lower than the control sample. This research was published in 1993 and is just one of many studies, which show beyond all reasonable doubt that providing nutritional supplements helps prevent cancer and stop cancer.

Antioxidants appear to boost the immune system and guard cells from free radical damage. They do this by binding to the sticky free radical's exposed electron, stopping it from attacking important cellular structures. A simple example of antioxidants at work is to take an apple and cut it in half; the air quickly attacks and oxidises the exposed apple, turning it brown. But if you cover one half in fresh lemon juice it will not turn brown. The lemon juice has acted as an antioxidant.

High doses of vitamin E stop cholesterol oxidation and rejuvenate the immune system in people over the age of 60 back almost to the level seen in young people.

There are many antioxidants together with many powerful vitamins and minerals that improve their functioning.

There are also several very clear and successful studies in the USA on the use of antioxidant megadoses to control existing cancers and prevent their recurrence.

Almost all the anti-ageing experts in the USA agree the following list of most beneficial supplements. I call them the 'magnificent six': beta-carotene, vitamin E, zinc, selenium, vitamin C and coenzyme Q 10.

(i) Beta-carotene and vitamin A

Beta-carotene is the precursor of vitamin A (or retinol) in the body. Vitamin A is crucial in the fight against cancer. There is a large volume of evidence providing a direct link between a low vitamin A level in the body and cancer. One such study, reported in 1993, followed 90,000 breast cancer patients in New England. Another, at the Sloan-Kettering Institute, Manhattan, linked supplementation of vitamin A to an 80 per cent remission rate in Leukaemia.

It is depressing how many health, nutrition and cancer books confuse beta-carotene and vitamin A. Vitamin A cannot be synthesised in the body and must be taken with food as retinol or in its precursor form beta-carotene. Whilst you can take vitamin A supplements (cod liver oil would be a good source) it is fat soluble and you should limit your dose. This is because excess vitamin A can be highly toxic and can cause your liver to be poisoned in its attempt to clean the excess out of the body. One friend, acting on misguided advice, took cod liver oil and evening primrose oil in large doses throughout a month and ended up turning a yellowish-grey! Far safer to take a little cod liver oil (max 1,000 mgs) whilst providing your body with good volumes of beta-carotene at the same time. The body only makes the amount of vitamin A that it needs from the beta-catotene, which is water-soluble so excess is quickly flushed from the body.

The first link between human cancer and low levels of vitamin A was in 1941 (Abelsetal) with low plasma levels being linked to gastro-intestinal cancers. Since that time there have been studies linking low vitamin A levels with cancers of the breast, prostate, stomach, colon/rectum and upper digestive tract.

If taken in correct doses, beta-carotene is claimed to cut cancer risk by up to 40 per cent. There are literally hundreds of studies on its efficacy in cancer prevention. (The only danger is for smokers where one study shows an increase in tumours by 13 per cent when the sample were smokers who then took beta-carotene.)

Beta-carotene is the orange pigment in carrots, peppers, apricots and pumpkins. You can also find it in sweet potato, chicory, spinach and kale.

It appears to mop up free radicals and block the proliferation of cancer cells.

Normal supplement amounts are 6 mgs, but anti-ageists recommend 10 mgs to 30 mgs (17,000 IU to 50,000 IU) and some take up to 50 mgs themselves. In one study amongst people with colon cancer 30 mgs per day caused cancer inhibition in 44 per cent of users after only two weeks. Dr Simin Meydani at Tufts studied the effects of 50 mg daily doses and showed that the natural immune system killer cells, which fight off cancer, were at much higher levels in the blood than in normal people.

Beta-carotene supplements should be taken with meals as the vitamin needs fat to help its absorption and it should be spread in two or three doses per day as it is easily eliminated from the body.

(ii) Vitamin E

The ultimate free radical buster!

It appears to inhibit the growth of cancer cells at the local level while at the global level protecting the immune system and particularly the B and T cells.

It is fat-soluble and stops the oxidisation of fats in the membranes of immune cells, brain cells and blood cells (think of it as stopping the membrane fats from turning rancid). Low intake of vitamin E has been linked to stomach cancer in one major Italian research study. It has also been shown to protect against lung cancer caused by pollution.

Vitamin E levels in green vegetables have particularly declined over the last 100 years due to soil depletion. A lettuce now contains one sixth of the vitamin E it had in 1900.

It can be found naturally in soya, nuts, seeds like pumpkin and sunflower, whole grains, whole wheat enriched flour, spinach and eggs. However it is important to note that from natural sources the most you are likely to ingest a day is only about 25–40 IU. Put out a bowl of organic pumpkin, sunflower and sesame seeds to nibble during the day (and throw away the packets of crisps and peanuts using hydrogenated oil).

Inorganic iron destroys vitamin E, while selenium helps it work. In turn, vitamin E helps vitamins A and C work.

About 60 per cent of the daily dose of vitamin E is expelled in the faeces so it needs to be constantly replaced. Take d-Alpha tocopherol (the d means its from natural sources) at a level of 400 IU, although some people recommend up to 1,000 IU.

Just to make life a little more complicated, there are several forms of vitamin E. Most available in the UK are tocopherol vitamin E's.

However, *America's Life Extension* magazine reported in spring 2002 that tocotrienol vitamin E has been shown to inhibit oestrogen positive receptor sites by as much as 50 per cent. Indeed they recorded that tocotrienol usage could cut tamoxifen requirements for women by 75 per cent.

Tocotrienols seem to collect in breast tissue (tocotrienol vitamin E is not in the EU approved list of medicines and so must be obtained from the USA).

(iii) Selenium

Selenium and vitamin E are synergistic, which means that they work better together than each on their own. Low selenium levels have been linked to cancer both of the stomach and breast. And the UK diet is the lowest in Europe for selenium intake, probably because of our soil, and our low consumption of garlic (garlic contains good levels of selenium). With vitamin E it helps protect against membrane damage; and it acts to replace certain harmful chemicals and heavy metals in the body, for example, mercury. Finally, selenium has an anti-viral and anti-bacterial action freeing up the immune system to fight off cancer.

In parts of China where the soil is rich in selenium, cancer has almost no presence, and there are estimates that a good selenium level in the body reduces cancer risk by 20 per cent.

Selenium is found in lobster, tuna fish, onions, broccoli, tomatoes, wheat germ and bran. Smoking, high intakes of polyunsaturated oils and fats and ingestion of mercury and lead cause a decline in its levels in the body. Fish oils contain quite good levels of selenium.

It is often claimed that eating two to three Brazil nuts per day provides your total requirement. Sadly there is a catch. The nuts must still be in their shells. Unshelled nuts come from a different area with low selenium and, in light, may have started to go rancid and become selenium depleted. But nuts in their shells come from an area quite high in radioactivity. So you just can't win!

Take the supplement but don't overdo it, as it is very powerful and not totally understood. The normal daily dose is 50–100 mcgs but you can go as high as, but not exceed, 200 mcgs.

(iv) Vitamin C

Linus Pauling, the pioneer of vitamin C, felt you should take 3–4 gms per day and up to 10 gms if you were ill. Nowadays there are claims about liver damage, and one study even claimed it caused cancer in excessive amounts, although there seem to be no confirmatory studies or categorical evidence for this. **Vitamin C is not recommended as a supplement in cases of brain tumours, as it can cause the spread of the tumour (asterocytosis).** However according to another study, women with breast cancer who take at least 10 gms of vitamin C live 16 times longer than those who don't.

Vitamin C seems to help strengthen cell membrane walls in the immune system, weaken cancer cell walls and neutralise aflatoxin (see section on parasites) amongst other more general healing and immune system benefits.

Neil Riordan (Aiden Clinic, Arizona) has published many articles on vitamin C (for example, *British Journal of Cancer* Vol 84, No. 11). He states that in his experience up to 46 per cent of cancer patients have scurvy or a lack of vitamin C.

Vitamin C brings about cell death in cancer cells; large doses cause the build up of hydrogen peroxide in cancer cells. Normal cells contain an enzyme, catalase which breaks this down, but cancer cells do not, resulting in their death. Lymphocytes in healthy people store large amounts of vitamin C ready to attack forming cancer cells.

He has also noted that several nutrients (quercetin, grape seed extract, biotin, vitamin K and lipoic acid) significantly promote the healing effects of vitamin C.

It is always better taken in the ester form as it is better for our stomachs than the straight ascorbic acid form.

Rosehips contain bioflavonoids and certain enzymes, which help assimilate vitamin C into the blood stream. Studies are currently underway on two citrus flavonoids (nobiletin and tangeretin) which substantially influence brain tumour invasion (ie the process of sending out rogue cells into secondary tissue such as the brain).

Vitamin C is water-soluble and passes through the body in about three hours, so it is best taken in smaller amounts at regular intervals or it time release capsules. It is particularly helpful in infection and healing and Dr Pauling actually found it would decrease infections by 25 per cent and cancers by 75 per cent if taken in 1–10 gm doses.

I have found one unsubstantiated claim that vitamin C should be not be taken when undergoing chemotherapy or radiotherapy, probably because it might protect the very cells the radiotherapy and chemotherapy are trying to kill off. It would seem wiser not to take high doses during these treatments.

The best natural sources are red peppers, berries, citrus fruits, green vegetables, cauliflower, sweet and normal potatoes and tomatoes.

When taking large amounts you should take magnesium to avoid kidney stones.

(v) Zinc

It is arguable that zinc per se is not an antioxidant but helps others do their job. It particularly helps the action of vitamin C and it works better itself when combined with vitamin A.

Zinc is credited with a vast number of things, from accelerating healing time to slowing the greying of hair and preventing white spots on fingernails. Zinc is very important for a healthy prostate gland and it is crucial in wound healing.

Alcoholics and people taking B-6 need higher amounts of zinc. It is found in meat, eggs, pumpkin seeds, sesame seeds, sunflower seeds and wheat germ and brewers yeast, shellfish and oysters.

Available as zinc sulphate or gluconate, 15–300 mgs can be taken, although recommended levels are 15–50 mgs.

Ingesting cow's milk and dairy products blocks the absorption of zinc. In children especially this depletes appetites and makes for 'picky eaters' so it is wrong to give milk to young children who do not eat a wide and varied diet on the basis that at least it is giving them nourishment. It actually prevents them from being nourished by restricting their appetites.

(vi) Coenzyme Q10 (CoQ10)

CoQ10 is a powerful antioxidant that, like vitamin E, protects the fats in membranes from being oxidised by free radicals. It helps stabilise all membranes.

CoQ10 also works inside the energy powerhouse (the mitochondria) in each and every cell in your body. Without it, exhaustion would set in and the immune system would collapse.

It is particlarly important as cancer cells have mitochondria that work abnormally, being unable to metabolise oxygen and producing energy only through a process called glycolysis. CoQ10 may well protect mitochondria from becoming abnormal.

In older people whose immune systems naturally decline with age, 60 mgs per day of CoQ10 produced antibody levels reaching those of young people.

CoQ10 can cross into the brain and is proven to prevent brain cell deterioration. Recent studies have shown an important role in prevention of dementia, and it can play an important role in patients with brain tumours.

It takes time to work, usually two to three months, and the normal dose is 30 mgs, although people with signs of chronic disease can take more. Studies show that the maximum level in the blood peaks with doses of 100 mgs. Like hormone supplementation, it should not be given to people under the age of 20 who should be producing more than enough anyway.

———

There are literally hundreds of antioxidants. Antioxidants abound in herbs and plants and many fruits and vegetables whilst some of the 'magnificent six' have many more bioflavonoids and cofactors that help their action. The more antioxidants you consume and the more diverse their source the more protected you are. Here are some others worth exploring:

(vii) Lycopene

Lycopene is another antioxidant found in yellow and orange vegetables, mostly tomatoes (especially cooked ones), strawberries, peppers, carrots and peaches. It actually binds to fats and lipids in the blood stream. The daily dose recommended is about 5–10 mgs. It is part of a package recommended to support a healthy prostate. The other effective ingredients are saw palmetto berries (oil) 150–400 mgs; Korean (panax) ginseng 3–5 mgs; pygeum bark (*Pygeum africans*) 1.5–2.0 mgs; zinc 15 mgs.

Prostate cancer is less common in vegetarians and in Asia where people eat more soya, vegetables, rice and less animal fats and dairy. Lycopene actually binds to fats and lipids in the body helping us overcome our Western diet. A Harvard study showed people with 10 plus servings of lycopene vegetables/fruits per week had 45 per cent less risk of cancer. In particular cooked tomatoes seem to release their lycopene more readily.

(viii) Lemon grass, kaffir lime and watercress

The Thais have more than their fair share of toxins around them but low, low cancer rates. Lemon grass, one of their natural and constant cooking herbs, is supposedly 100 times stronger then beta-carotene as an antioxidant, galanga and kaffir lime leaves are three to five times stronger. Back in the UK watercress, beet-root and a number of natural fresh organic herbs also help boost the immune system more than most vitamin pills.

(ix) Circuminoids

These are phytochemical phenol products that have broad and powerful antioxidant benefits and act both to bind to free radicals and prevent their formation in the first place. They work particularly well in conjunction with vitamin E and are found as the yellow pigment of tumeric. Curcumin causes cell death in melanoma cells and several types of cancer cells in laboratory tests.

(x) Grape seed extract and pine bark

Both these substances contain OPCs (oligomeric proanthocyanidins), although they each contain slightly different co-factors. OPCs are very powerful antioxidants, reputedly 20–50 times more powerful than vitamins E and C. OPCs prevent the oxidation process that forms free radicals at the cellular level, and scavenge free radicals throughout the body. Their power as an anti-cancer agent is being researched currently.

Q17. What other supplements might help?

(i) Multivitamin and mineral supplements.

Almost all the top anti-ageing experts in the USA take a good multivitamin and mineral supplement daily. There are some questions over the benefit of iron (and actually quite a lot of concern) and problems with its absorption. Look for supplements that are iron free, or contain organic iron. However the real benefit is in trace but important minerals like boron, magnesium, calcium, phosphorus and manganese. Multivitamins tend to provide poor levels of beta-carotene, vitamins C and E although good levels of certain B vitamins.

One of the biggest problems with all vitamin supplements and especially multivitamins is the poor absorption rates of pills. It is estimated that up to 85 per cent of a multivitamin pill can pass straight through you. Look for colloidal supplements, which are more readily absorbed. The problem of absorption is further worsened for vitamins such as C and beta-carotene, which can be flushed out of the body in less than three hours, as they are water-soluble. There is some debate as to whether any of the C or beta-carotene even reaches the more distant cells of your body. It is better to take small doses of these vitamins frequently in an attempt to keep your cellular system topped up.

(ii) B vitamins

B complex often contains a number of individual B vitamins, which are potent when mixed together rather than used separately. Beware though, that some B complex are yeast based pills and you would be wise to avoid these.

Cooking particularly destroys B vitamins, as does alcohol, caffeine, food processing, the pill (oestrogen) and smoking. A lot of athletes have B deficiency because it is expelled in sweat, being water-soluble

B vitamins particularly help in the nervous system and with cell growth, memory and red blood cell production. B-1, B-2, B-6, and B-12 are essential to the body, whilst low levels of B-2, B-3 and especially B-12 have been linked to cancer. All of these may be found in multivitamin or B complex supplements. But there are others, which are important to consider but not always found in these forms. These are:

- Biotin – essential for vitamin C to work. Good sources are nuts, egg yolk (but egg white destroys it), organic complete rice, fruits and milk. Take 0.3 mgs per day especially if you are on antibiotics.
- Folic acid – critical for the accurate replication of DNA, your genetic code, every time cells divide. It is found in green leafy vegetables, egg yolk, liver, pumpkin, apricots, avocado, carrots and beans and whole grain flour. For cancer prevention, take 400 mcgs per day (never more than 800 mcgs). It is essential at the very point of cancer formation because when DNA divides, mutations can occur and folic acid reduces the risk. It is also crucial for cancer sufferers during radiotherapy treatment. Folic acid helps reduce the risk of colon cancer and is also important in retaining memory as you age.
- Inositol and choline – two separate B vitamins, but they work together. They are crucial for healthy membranes, the immune system (where they aid the work of vitamin E), and they are two of the few substances to cross the blood brain barrier and go into brain cells aiding memory. (Choline is now thought to help stave off Alzheimer's.) Enemies are alcohol, the pill and caffeine.

  The best natural sources are liver, beans, egg yolks, offal, wheat germ and cabbage. But soya lecithin provides both. Daily doses are inositol 250–500 mgs, choline 500–1000 mgs. Take soya lecithin (from soya beans) in capsules (up to 3 gms per day, maximum) or in powder sprinkled over your breakfast cereal. Inositol and choline help keep the liver from being clogged up with fats and thus are very effective in this area of the immune system.
- B-17 (laetrile or amygdalin) – this is a naturally occurring vitamin identified in 1955 by Ernst Krebs and claimed to be extremely effective in the treatment of cancer or simply in prevention. Its use is controversial because the Federal Drug Administration (FDA) in the USA has not approved it (although why they officially needed to approve a naturally

occurring vitamin in the first place is a mystery in itself). A Senate committee (often accused of being biased and with rumoured drug industry connections) seemed unimpressed by evidence that:

- Three quarters of 80 cancer test patients had seen their cancer tumours go or reduce in size
- Populations where B-17 is naturally consumed are cancer free (eg Hunzaland/Nepal. Mind you, they probably don't have too many mobile phones, processed foods and pesticides in Nepal either!)
- The argument runs that 100 years ago we naturally ate far more B-17. It can be found naturally in apricot kernels, apple seeds and peach kernels where it can reach the 3 per cent level, plus the seeds of prunes, plums and cherries, and in walnuts, brazils, cashews, macadamia nuts, millet, buckwheat and cranberries and cranberry juice. The higher the level of B-17 in the kernels the more bitter their taste.

The controversy centres on the fact that B-17 can been broken down to form cyanide and is thus dangerous.

This needs further examination. As we said in Q4 the power stations, or mitochondria, are different in cancer cells. They don't use oxygen but burn the sugars using an enzyme called glucosidase.

This enzyme turns B-17 into benzaldehyde (an analgesic) and hydrogen cyanide (a poison), thus killing the cell.

Normal cells produce energy using oxygen and an enzyme rhodinase. Rhodinase neutralises B-17.

To put this in context a cancer cell has 3,000 times the glucosidase of a normal cell ensuring that, inside those cells, benzaldehyde and hydrogen cyanide are made in dangerous quantities. So B-17 is like a natural 'search and destroy' homing device for cancer cells.

Clinics using B-17 treatments (along with vitamin megadoses) have been forced out of America across the border into Mexico. It is illegal in California, for example, to recommend any cancer treatment other than surgery, radiotherapy, and chemotherapy. This furthers their dangerous quack image, casting a shadow over the vitamin and stopping proper research. Conversely, disciples of B-17 claim that the pharmaceutical companies are trying to protect the huge profits they make by restricting treatments to ineffective but profitable chemotherapy drugs. Impasse.

According to *Nutrition Almanac* in the USA five to 35 apricot kernels eaten throughout the day can be a sufficient preventative amount; but people are advised never to eat more than five at one time. Krebs himself recommended taking 10 seeds per day for life.

Tablets or vitamin pills can be obtained and two to four tablets each of 100 mgs is the suggested daily preventative amount. Treatment clinics for cancer patients use both apricot kernels and doses of four to six 500 mgs tablets per day. Tests show cumulative amounts of around 3 gms can be digested safely but it is recommended that no more than 1 gm is taken at any one time.

Great care has to be taken with people undergoing B-17 treatment or metabolic therapy treatment. The by-products of B-17 breakdown and its action will pass to the liver where they in turn are rendered harmless by an enzyme, glucuronide. However, firstly, everybody's levels of this enzyme are different and, secondly, in cancer patients the liver function is likely to be impaired and levels of this enzyme might be low and insufficient to deal with the B-17 action.

B-17 action is supported and enhanced by two protein digestive enzymes; one from pineapple (bromelain), one from papaya (papain).

The two enzymes help to de-mask the outer shield of the malignant cell and although the two enzymes can be taken in pill form it is probably better to eat a pineapple and two papayas, if you can manage it every day!

B-17 is also enhanced in its action by taking 5–6 gms of vitamin C, plus vitamins E and A. Successes with B-17 have involved all these supplements and some critics claim it is these 'extras' that are the real successes.

In Britain, Canada, Italy, Mexico, Belgium and the USA oncologists in clinics are currently using B-17 as part of 'dynamic metabolic therapy' and they claim to have good success rates, although there are a few cast iron statistical studies with humans. But on 25 August 2000, the USA FDA and Department of Justice instructed two companies selling laetrile to stop supplying it beyond their individual state borders, effectively shutting down their businesses. According to the FDA the status of laetrile is, 'no different than that of any other unapproved drug.'

The curious thing is that this ban extended to the supply of apricot kernels as well! You can, of course, buy apricots anywhere and crack the kernels open yourself and B-17 is available in certain European countries and supposedly even on the German NHS, although I haven't personally checked this.

The US Government has now also banned the planting of bitter almond trees, so they seem unequivocal in their pursuit of B-17. All this from a Government that allows melatonin and other hormones to be freely sold in their supermarkets.

(iii) Calcium and vitamin D

Low calcium causes a hormone calcitrol to be produced, which enhances fat storage and fat stores more toxins, as I covered earlier. Hence it is important in cancer prevention. Some studies have shown that depleted levels of calcium are linked to breast and colon cancers.

Although the majority of us get more than enough calcium without eating dairy products, talk of brittle bones later on in life has focused more attention on it. In fact the issue with calcium is not intake levels but storage and loss levels from the body. It is easily absorbed, stored and highly reusable as long as vitamin D (particularly D-3) and magnesium are plentiful. Resistance training will cause more of it to be taken into the bones and improve density. But smoking, oestrogen and alcohol, for example, deplete stores significantly.

Controversially, milk and dairy products can also accelerate the rate at which calcium is lost from the body! Dairy products, apart from containing hormones, pesticides, and trace metals, block the body's ability to absorb zinc and iron and this in turn greatly imbalances magnesium levels affecting the storage levels. Coral calcium and coral kelp are good non-dairy sources of calcium, magnesium and a host of other minerals.

They are currently favoured as cancer fighting supplements in the alternative field as they have an alkalising effect and so help to balance the body's pH. Since both are natural products they have all their minerals in an organic and bioavailable form. Okinawans (see later under calorie restriction and cancer reduction) consume vast amounts of minerals from the nearby coral leaching into their food chain.

Vitamin D itself has a strong anti-cancer role even though it is only present in small quantities in our food. It significantly affects the incidence of prostate cancer.

Vitamin D has a molecular structure similar to steroids, in fact cholesterol is a precursor for both. Sunlight acts on the skin causing the photo-conversion of a form of cholesterol into vitamin D-3. However short days, heavy clothing, office working and polluted cities can make people vitamin D deficient. There is evidence that black people's skin pigmentation prevents vitamin D being made in this way, and this fact is being linked to their increased rates of prostate cancer, for example.

In May 2002, The Howard Hayes Medical Institute heard how vitamin D protects against colon cancer.

Apart from regulating calcium metabolism, it stimulates its absorption from food and plays a wider role in general mineral metabolism.

A good source of vitamin D is fish oil (but not cod liver oil). Herring, sprat and tuna are good sources. High protein and high calcium intake inhibit vitamin D.

Q18. What hormone supplements might help?

Hormones are very, very potent chemicals and, under normal healthy conditions, they are in complete balance in your body. This is called homeostasis. However, it is easy to throw that balance out by eating or drinking 'sugar', by stress, lack of sleep or by absorption of outside hormones. Those that you take in from outside sources tend to be pretty dangerous; those that you make yourself are crucial. A couple of them in particular are powerful cleansers or neutralisers of free radicals in your body. Although none in the UK is available as a supplement except on prescription, many are available at health food and vitamin stores in the USA. Extreme caution is recommended before taking any of them and a conversation with a knowledgeable doctor is essential.

(i) Melatonin

Melatonin is primarily produced in the pineal gland deep inside the brain. However, recently it has also been found produced in the gut and retina. In the pineal it is produced when we sleep and it is directly linked to how well we sleep. The peak of production is usually about one to two hours after falling asleep and it pushes you into a deeper level of sleep. However, levels of production decline markedly as we age to almost nil at the age of 70. (This explains in part why older people sleep less well.) Sleeping with the light on disrupts melatonin production, as does long-haul flying and night shift work. A recent study shows that women who work night shifts have a higher breast cancer rate and it is thought that this is due to their lowered levels of melatonin.

It is made from an essential (ie one we can't make ourselves and have to eat) amino acid called tryptophan, which is first converted to seratonin, a brain chemical associated with mood, and then to melatonin.

Melatonin is very powerful and is perhaps the only antioxidant capable of entering every cell in the body and neutralising all free radicals. One of the key glands it stimulates is the thymus, which plays a core role in the immune system, being the store of T cells.

The thymus degenerates by 90 per cent as we get older, reducing dramatically the potency of our immune system. In tests with cancer patients 10 mgs of melatonin per night produced a marked improvement in immune systems, in particular improving levels of interferon-gamma, T cells and interleukin-2, which is a hormone that aids T cell production.

Breast cancer patients have low levels of melatonin and melatonin use has been found to have a positive effect with breast, prostate and lung cancer. It seems to work best with solid tumours rather than metastasised ones, or those in brain or liver. Normal doses are 3–10 mgs. Some treatments go to 40 mgs although there are dangers of hallucination above 10 mgs. Because it is so powerful it should not be taken for long periods. Melatonin is naturally produced in good quantities until puberty and it should never be given to children. You cannot buy it in the UK, and it is available only on prescription.

(ii) Human growth hormone (Hgh)

Human growth hormone, or somatotropin, is a simple protein produced by the pituitary gland. It is also produced during sleep and again is found primarily in children pre-puberty. It passes into the bloodstream to the liver where it is converted to growth factors DGF 1 & 2, which carry the message to other parts of the body.

Its primary function is to help bones grow and to assist in the transport and utilisation of amino acids, the components of protein. In tests using injections of Hgh with adults, the hormone was shown to reduce fatty tissue and promote lean muscle mass.

It does seem to play an anti-cancer role but this is imprecise and certainly injections of Hgh in adults are not without side effects. Like melatonin, Hgh production falls dramatically with age. Its action seems to be that it is essential to the immune system by producing superoxide radicals. These activate the macrophages that seek and destroy infecting rogue cells. Melatonin itself may increase Hgh levels.

The amino acid argenine has been shown to stimulate the pituitary to produce Hgh, as has ornithine and, indirectly, choline.

Taking these three supplements has been recommended for

increasing Hgh production. The other effective stimulator appears to be exercise, and particularly resistance training, where muscles are deliberately fatigued by heavier than normal weights. Lower body workouts are particularly effective.

Finally, a calorie-restricted diet also produces higher than normal levels of Hgh.

(iii) DHEA (Dehydroepiandrosterone)

DHEA requires healthy kidneys (and adrenal glands) for its production. It particularly helps the immune system to recognise infecting bacteria, viruses and cancer cells. It seems to stimulate T cell and IL-2 production by protecting the thymus from decline.

It is one of the most abundant hormones in our bodies when we are younger but, again, levels lower significantly as we age and the adrenal glands get smaller.

It is widely believed that a person's risk of cancer may be correlated with the levels of DHEA in the blood or urine. However, to date, opinions are mixed and there is even a little evidence that taking DHEA may promote some cancers causing an increased risk of, for example, prostate or breast tumours. Conversely, several recent studies do show its importance overall in the anti-cancer fight.

DHEA replacement therapy is available in the USA and although people do take it, it really seems to be an imprecise science at the moment. You cannot buy the tablets in the UK, only in the USA.

One suggestion I came across was to take a DHEA precursor, which is found in wild yam, as this would at least allow the body some control over the DHEA levels subsequently produced. (Wild yam, primarily found in China and Japan, is reported to help boost the immune system and overall health.)

Q19. Are there any other important hormones that play an anti-cancer role?

Yes, eicosanoids

Many people, including doctors, have never heard of eicosanoids, although they may have heard of one of their subgroups, prostaglandins. In fact, although eicosanoids have been the subject of Nobel Prizes (Sir Richard Vane, in the late 70s), they have been widely ignored.

Eicosanoids are hormones; very, very powerful ones, produced by each and every one of your cells, not by endocrine glands. There are over 100 of them. Because they do not need to travel round the body they don't last long, working and self-destructing in a matter of seconds. This makes analysing them very difficult. Basically they react to the messages provided by the hormones, toxins and nutrients in the fluid around the cell and then activate receptor sites on the surface of the cell to tell it what to do. Some are good and work to protect the cell, some are bad and make matters worse.

What is interesting about them is that you can influence whether you make more good ones or bad ones. Although there are a number of influencing factors, the three most relevant to this book are:

- Consumption of EPA, eg in fish oils
- Levels of insulin in the body
- Levels of stress hormones.

Fish oils

Grandma's favourite, cod liver oil, really does work. Indeed, oily fish are a very rich source of a substance called EPA, which is an example of a long-chained omega 3 fatty acid. This has a profound protective effect on the body in many areas. (Some seed oils contain omega 3, however these are short chained omega 3 fatty acids and seem to have a neutral effect in the body.)

Much has been written about 'good' omega 3 fatty acids and

'bad' omega 6 fatty acids. Long ago when we hunted from our caves they were probably in the ratio of one to one in our bodies and even 100 years ago they were one to two. Now the average New Yorker has a ratio of one to 25 (good to bad)

EPA and GLA (a substance from evening primrose or borage oil) are converted into stores of DGLA. But, unfortunately, even nasty old hydrogenated oils can raise the DGLA levels in the body.

The problem comes because DGLA can be used to make any one of the 100 eicosanoids, good or bad. And what determines the production of bad eicosanoids is the activity of just one enzyme. Crucially, DGLA is converted by this enzyme into arachidonic acid, which in turn makes only bad eicosanoids such as prostaglandins.

EPA from fish oil blocks this enzyme thus ensuring the balance shifts away from bad towards good eicosanoid production. Only EPA can block this enzyme; evening primrose oil and borage or hydrogenated fats cannot.

All 60 trillion of your body's cells can and do make eicosanoids, so clearly the preponderance of good guys to bad guys is crucial. Those people who take evening primrose oil (eg for period pains), should be careful and think seriously about taking a fish oil supplement as well. But remember, because fish oils are high in vitamin A which has a toxic effect on the liver if taken in excess, you should limit your supplement to 1,000 mgs per day.

Levels of insulin in the body

Insulin stimulates the enzyme that makes bad eicosanoids. This has implications for overweight people, who often flood their bodies with carbohydrates and sugars and thus stimulate excess insulin production.

Levels of stress hormones

Cortisol and steroids, for example, are also known to have a stimulating effect on this same enzyme. Both are produced by the endocrine glands in response to stimuli from the brain. So eicosanoids are the final link in the chain between brain moods and your cellular biochemistry. Negative thoughts, stress and guilt are all factors that switch on bad eicosanoid production through this link with the endocrine system, bathing the localised cellular system in a negative environment.

Other factors

Other substances referred to elsewhere in this book are linked to eicosanoids and their action. Ginger contains sequiterpenes, which inhibit the production of bad eicosanoids (especially prostaglandins and leukotrienes).

In garlic there is a substance called ajoene which limits bad eicosanoid responses and, in turn, has been shown to reduce blood pressure, inflammation, and inhibit cancers.

The original eicosanoid research 20 years ago studied the effect of aspirin (salicylate) in blocking bad eicosanoid production. The Mayo clinic has confirmed this research and showed how just 81 mgs of aspirin per day could reduce cancer risks. They also reconfirmed the effectiveness of omega 3.

So although this work still needs the finishing touches, there is already strong evidence that eicosanoids have a critical bearing on cellular biochemistry and thus on the cancer potential there.

It cannot be stressed enough that hormones are very, very powerful. Powerful enough to 'trump' anything else in and around the cell.

Q20. What natural herbal or plant supplements might help?

Herbs have been used to treat ailments for thousands of years. The rose gardens surrounding Hampton Court Palace were in fact herb gardens in the middle ages, whilst red clover blossoms were a herb of choice for Hippocrates. Sadly, the get well quick mentality of recent decades has seen many long established herbs with proven track records dropped in favour of, for example, antibiotics.

When it comes to cancer treatments, modern medicine contains a huge paradox, especially for the cancer sufferer. Namely at the very moment one needs one's immune system in tip-top order, many of the medical profession's cancer treatments are in fact weakening or destroying it. Sometimes Biological Response Modifiers (BRMs) are given to patients along with the chemotherapy drugs to reduce the side effects and damage to the immune system.

Some natural supplements can have the same desired effect, reducing the damage to the sufferer's immune system or, in the case of the non-sufferer, boosting the whole immune response and actually increasing the odds that this person will not become a cancer sufferer in the first place.

Two common BRM's are often given with cancer treatments. These are hormone-like products called cytokines:

- Interleukins, that stimulate the production of white blood cells
- Interferons, that help the body produce antiviral chemicals and stimulate the destruction of foreign bodies(by stimulating macrophage production).

Much interest in the medical laboratories now centres on natural herbal cytokines, which seem to produce strong immune responses without the side effects.

Whether or not you have cancer the herbal supplements you might consider using are:

(i) Astragalus

Astragalus (*Astragalus membranaceous*) has been around in Chinese medicine for two thousand years. It is known as haung

93

qi, or chi, because it was thought to boost natural body energy and is taken from the root of a plant needing four to seven years to mature. This herb has been used as an immune system booster and specifically to treat burns, abscesses, and for hepatitis. In Chinese hospitals it is now used to help people recover from the negative effects of radiotherapy and chemotherapy.

Its wide usage in China, because it offers a direct boost to the immune system, has been supported by recent tests in the US and has led the medical profession to conclude it does have benefits in the fight against cancer. It is soon to be granted FDA approval as an anti-cancer agent. In tests at the Hiroshima School of Medicine in Japan, it was shown to directly increase B-lymphocyte growth, T cell, interlukin and antibody production. It seems to have the added benefit of improving the effectiveness of radiotherapy by boosting the cancer fighting system.

Researchers in the USA reported that cancer patients undergoing radiotherapy had twice the survival rates if they took astragalus, and all of the above has been confirmed by the University of Texas.

Astragalus appears to contain bioflavonoids, choline and a polysaccharide, astragalan B. The latter controls bacterial infection and viruses by binding to their outer membranes and weakening them. It is also an important adjunct now in the fight against Aids.

It should be taken with meals, three times per day with a total intake of around 2,000–3,000 mgs per day.

(ii) Garlic

Garlic (*Allium sativum*) is antibacterial and antiviral, it actively boosts the immune system and people who eat garlic contract less cancers. People who eat garlic more than once per week have half the rate of colon cancer in a study of 42,000 older women in Iowa. And prostate cells exposed to the garlic chemical SAMC grow at only 25 per cent the normal rate. Garlic has been shown to inhibit cancer in all tissues including breast, liver and colon. It should be eaten crushed or raw because cooking destroys its active ingredients. (Take out the green centre and ideally buy it fresh when it is not made up of obvious concentric leaves, and your breath won't smell!)

Garlic is probably most talked about for its ingredient allicin, which actually prevents cancer cell proliferation. Together with other natural flavones it seems to help the immune system by its third party work, like lowering blood pressure and cholesterol levels, whilst exhibiting antiviral and antibacterial activities (eg in helping cut yeast and mould infections in the body). Garlic contains good levels of tryptophan, the precursor of seratonin, which is the precursor of melatonin.

Few people mention its selenium and germamium contents, when both are such good strengthening agents in the fight against cancer. They mop up free radicals and, along with the S-ally cysteine and Dialyl-sulphide also found in garlic, they neutralise carcinogens. Germamium appears to help transport oxygen into cancer cells. Cancer cells hate oxygen: they cannot metabolise it and so they die. It also helps the body produce higher levels of interferon, a powerful anti-cancer force.

Garlic's action with moulds and yeast also extends to its abilities to neutralise aflatoxins, which they and parasites produce. Research (Soni KB 1997) has shown that garlic enhances a liver enzyme that helps to detoxify aflatoxins before they cause damage.

Garlic also seems to have an effect in protecting the body against the side effects of radiotherapy, particularly from DNA and chromosome damage. Finally, doses of garlic seem to directly inhibit bladder and stomach cancer tumour growth

Onions, chives and leeks also have similar, but lesser, benefits.

iii) Noni juice

Sadly the heavy marketing of this product, often bordering on the over claim, gets in the way of the real and excellent benefits of this natural fruit. I am a firm personal convert. It can be eaten as a fruit but is far more readily available as a concentrated fruit drink.

Firstly, it helps combat acid ash in the body, helping it achieve an alkaline pH, which is beneficial to all cellular biochemistry, and particularly the immune system in the fight against cancer.

Secondly, it has been shown in extensive research to promote a stronger immune system increasing the production of both B and T lymphocytes and to be a 'protector' against cancer.

Noni contains a number of very potent alkaloids. Bromelain is known to weaken the walls of cancer cells, xeronine seems to help repair cells and in tests it produces a strong immune response against cancer cells. Noni is full of alkaloids and phyto-chemicals and Dr D L Davis, the senior science advisor to the US Public Health Service is very clear that, 'phytochemicals can take tumours and diffuse them'.

The Thais take it to aid digestion and avoid bacteria in the stomach and it can also be used to heal wounds and minor skin problems.

iv) Pau d'Arco

Pau d'Arco comes from the bark of a South American tree and has some anti-cancer activity due to the ingredient lapachol. It is a very powerful agent and originally was thought to have many direct effects on cancer. Due to the 20 or more active ingredients making it effective as an anti-fungal, antiviral, antibacterial and antimicrobial agent, it is now thought to be a very powerful, all-round body cleanser. This takes the pressure off the immune system so that the body can better restore full immune system power to fight the cancer.

It is widely used as a natural agent against parasites and candida and thus frees up the immune system to act fully in other areas.

v) Black cumin (*Nigella sativa*)

This is sometimes called cinnamon flower or nutmeg flower and is used for a variety of illnesses particularly in the Middle East. Studies in 1991 by Nair showed extracts from the seeds to be toxic to cancer cells.

White blood cells treated with nigella seeds produce higher levels of interleukin plus a specific factor that stops the growth of tumours. Indeed two studies in 1997 and 1998, one by Medenica in the South Carolina, Immuno-Biology Research Laboratory and the other by Worthen both showed that the seeds inhibited tumour growth and the blood supply growth necessary for a tumour to form.

(vi) Essiac (sometimes called Cassie tea)

Sadly, this product, or rather blend of ingredients, is surrounded in mythology that tends to overshadow its real powers.

It was probably used by native American Indians for several hundred years as a herbal remedy in all sorts of illnesses. In 1922 a patient of Nurse Rene Caisse in Canada told her about a herbal infusion that had cured her breast cancer some 20 years before. Caisse saw the results for herself and incorporated the use of the remedy into her patients' treatments.

Over the following 50 or more years Rene Caisse ran a very successful free cancer clinic in Canada, then another in conjunction with several doctors, notably Dr Charles Brusch in New England. Although she had clinical X-rays and pathological proof of her results, the Canadian Government never officially approved the treatment. Her own view was that, 'if it doesn't actually cure cancer, it does afford significant relief.'

She treated her own 72 year old mother with the tea under the supervision of Dr Roscoe Graham, consultant and specialist. The tea was administered 12 times a day for 10 days, and her mother lived to 90 years of age.

The active ingredients were:

- **Burdock root** – a well known blood purifier which can decrease cell mutation and inhibit tumours. It has a reasonably high selenium content
- **Sheep sorrel** – a traditional and powerful Indian remedy for everything from eczema to ringworm; it does have an effect in herpes, ulcers and cancer seemingly by stimulating the endocrine system. It needs to be prepared slowly and correctly to be effective.
- **Slippery elm** – calcium, magnesium and vitamin rich, it has a healing effect on the lungs and internal organs. It also helps reduce acid ash in the body.
- **Indian rhubarb** – very cleansing to the liver and intestinal system. It also helps transport oxygen throughout the body and has an antibiotic and anti-yeast action and reduces inflammation. In 1980 studies showed that it also had a clear anti-tumour effect.

Whilst working with Dr Brusch between 1959 and 1978, Nurse Caisse added four other herbs to the formula (the current formula is her name spelled backwards). The four additions are:

- **Watercress** – a powerful antioxidant, containing bioflavonoids; it is a good blood purifier.
- **Blessed thistle** – a blood purifier and immune booster
- **Red clover** – the herb of Hippocrates, the flowers are currently undergoing tests in the UK for breast cancer control.
- **Kelp** – like chlorophyll and spyrogina, kelp is a strong provider of natural minerals especially iron and calcium in an organic and easily assimilated form. Kelp is antibacterial and sea vegetables, in general, help reduce acidity in the body thus improving immune function.

Nurse Caisse recommended 12–13 cups of the infusion per day. Shortly before she died she sold the 'secret' formula to a company called Resperin.

(vii) Echinacea

Originally in the 16th and 17th centuries, echinacea was used by native Americans for just about every medical need. This flower has a number of active ingredients but its usage was surpassed by antibiotics, although it is now having a renaissance as an immune booster against colds and flu.

Echinacea (or purple coneflower) is a native plant to America and was first used officially in medical practices in 1887. Most researched in Germany, it boosts the immune system directly and particularly aids the ingestion of foreign particles by the white cells. It also directly attacks viruses. Whilst it is most used for helping in infections of the upper respiratory tract (eg colds, where it helps both prevent and shorten the duration), it does have several anti-cancer benefits.

It can reduce secondary infection after radiotherapy and chemotherapy. There is also some evidence that it helps reduce the rate of growth of brain tumours and it appears (according to the University of Munich) to stimulate interleukin and the production of white cells, increasing both T and B lymphocytes, the former by 30 per cent. Another study showed that it has a direct effect on interferon production, which in turn disrupts the genetic code of foreign particles like viruses and probably even cancer cells.

Whilst it does strengthen the immune system it should not be taken in the long term as it thins the blood. Six to eight weeks is the recommended maximum period.

In a paper by M J Verhoef (1999) *Neurology* vol. 52, echinacea was studied as an alternative therapy for neurological disease and in brain tumour patients with some successful results. 1,200 mgs is a normal daily dose.

(viii) Green tea

You should drink green tea every day. It contains many anti-oxidant polyphenols, especially catechins, which have been shown to inhibit the spread of cancer (*Nature* 1997; Jankun).

Green tea seems to have a positive effect with people on radio-therapy and chemotherapy. It has also emerged as a leading candidate for the prevention of UV-induced skin cancer. And, if that's not enough, apparently green tea also helps you slim and evens out skin tone and wrinkles!

(ix) Ginseng

Ginseng has energy inducing properties some of which come from its caffeine content. However it does have cancer benefits.

There are essentially two different types of ginseng, of which the first seems to be the more relevant in cancer treatment. The two types are:

* *Panax:* Oriental, Asiatic, Chinese, Korean or Japanese
* *Siberian:* a completely different plant.

Ginseng (*Panax*) stimulates the production of interleukin and boosts B and T lymphocytes and macrophages. There is some evidence that it boosts spleen cells to become active killers of cancer cells. In mice with lung cancer it reduces tumours by 44 per cent.

It also plays a part in relieving and preventing prostate cancer. Ginseng (*Panax*) should not be taken during radiotherapy or chemotherapy because it can result in decreased blood platelet clotting and bleeding.

(x) Cat's claw (Uno de Gato)

Alkaloids are powerful substances found in certain herbs and plants. There are six such oxindole alkaloids in Uno de Gato bark.

This natural substance is found mainly in the Peruvian Rain Forest and China. It is known to be antiviral, anti-inflammatory, an antioxidant and an immune stimulator. Four of the alkaloids in particular help in phagocytosis, attacking, wrapping up and removing harmful organisms, viruses, antigens and rogue cells.

The herb has been shown to be very powerful in its use with both cancer and Aids, and it is very beneficial in relieving side effects from both radio and chemotherapy.

You should take 1 gm per day on an empty stomach. It can also be drunk as a tea using 300 mgs per cup.

As an anti-cancer aid it is combined with wild yam and aloe vera, the combination being a very strong antiviral, anti-bacterial force and having a very strong synergistic effect on the immune system.

(xi) Salycylic acid

You may know this best as aspirin. But you don't have to take pills, you can eat almonds, for example. In the 19th century people used to chew willow bark because of its anti-inflammatory benefits.

The Mayo Clinic in 2000 showed that 81 mgs of aspirin per day (about a sixth of one tablet) could cut cancer rates (eg prostate, colon) by 40 to 50 per cent.

Aspirin has had several good reviews in studies in the last two years. Its anti-inflammatory activities reduce the size of intestinal polyps (precursors to colon cancer) and reduce the size of enlarged prostates.

Q21. Are there any other dietary factors that might help prevent or control a cancer?

All of the following help in the fight against cancer:

(i) Soy or soya

In July 2002 Cancer Research UK published findings on the clear benefits of soya. A study involving two pieces of research, the US National Cancer Institute and the University of Singapore concluded that women who consumed the most soya were 60 per cent less likely to have risky, dense breast tissue than those consuming little soya.

Soya contains substances that are positive cancer protectors. Chemicals called phytoestrogens in soya actually block the effect of animal oestrogen in breast and prostate cancers by blocking receptors on the cell surface where oestrogen can alight and promote cancer growth. The anti-breast cancer drug Tamoxifen acts in the same way, but has notable side effects. The receptors on the cell surface will accept any oestrogen, animal or plant. Phytoestrogens are also found more generally in many other plants and may be called isoflavones.

One soya isoflavone, genistein, has been specifically shown to block mammary tumours in animals, and also to prevent the growth of the blood supply to all tumours. (This blood supply is essential for a tumour's growth.) Asian women can have up to 1,000 times more genistein in their blood than Western women. There is evidence that soya can repair sun damage and lighten pigmentation spots.

Soya should ideally be organically grown and non-GM. Avoid soya products like mass-produced soy sauce because of the additives it contains and look for miso soup, tofu and tempeh. Soya milk and yoghurts can be bought in health food shops and consumed instead of milk and milk yoghurts. Soya protein can be used instead of meat and miso soup is high in the anti-cancer health food list. Soya beans themselves are a terrific source of vitamin E.

It is estimated that the equivalent of two and a half bowls of soya milk per day provides a start level for strengthening and protection, but 30–100 gms per day is the ideal amount. You can supplement further with soya isoflavones in capsules.

The question everybody has to ask themselves is, 'why use milk, which has severe question marks hanging over it, when soya is actually a cancer protector?' The majority of people in the world do not use dairy products, or use them sparingly, so on a volume basis, milk is actually a substitute for soya in the world, not the other way round!

Soya does have its critics but most seem factually inaccurate.

It is claimed that soya contains 10 times the aluminium of milk; this is not true, they are roughly the same. It is linked to allergies, particularly child allergies, but then so is milk and all the 'evidence' seems anecdotal. It is claimed that consumption is actually very limited in the Far East and contains increased levels of phylic acid. Another generalisation. Anyone who has travelled there will know that beans are regularly consumed and a regular Chinese breakfast is rice in soya milk. Finally, people site the Gerson Institute who do not recommend it. I spoke with Charlotte Gerson about this. In the original Gerson treatment soya was frowned upon because it contains loads of phytic acid and phytic acid can block mineral absorption, the very cornerstone of the Gerson Therapy (see Q24). They also avoid pulses and green beans for this reason. Interestingly the Plaskett therapy which updates and modernises Gerson from a scientific nutritional and biochemical basis does use some soya.

The real case to answer is the possible link to allergies in the West and the fact that soya is an incomplete protein containing, for example, no B-12 which needs to be provided by other sources.

Another generalism is that it is a non-argument to suggest that high soya consumption in the Far East is linked to low cancer rates. Curiously many of the same people argue that the consumption of B-17 by Hunzas is uniquely linked to their low cancer rates!

Clearly the truth is that soya consumption is just a part of a diet that contains many vegetables and rice. The sensible solution is to understand that you cannot simply bring one element of a Far East diet to the West and expect it to 'work'. But it might just help!

(ii) Other isoflavones

Beans, lentils, chickpeas, many vegetables and legumes all contain good levels of isoflavones as do herbs such as red clover blossoms, which were used by many ancient herbalists. Tests are currently taking place at The Royal Marsden Hospital to see if red clover can actually prevent breast cancer.

These foods are not just important for their phytoestrogen but the fact that their fibre content in the gut actually aids the disposal of, for example, excess oestrogen hormone from the body. In 1900 up to 30 per cent of protein in the British diet came from pulses (beans, peas, lentils). Now it is less than 2 per cent. We are no longer eating foods that best protect us.

(iii) Fish oils

Fish oils contain vitamin A, vitamin D and high levels of long chain omega 3 fatty acids, as covered in the piece on eicosanoids. They are the ultimate 'triple whammy' in the fight against cancer. However, all fish oils were not created equal. Cod liver oil has the highest levels of omega 3 but little vitamin D. Perhaps you should mix cod liver oil and general fish oils, or at least read the labels! Although oils generally tend to encourage cancer development, omega 3 seems to stop the spread of cancer cells, probably by binding to cell membranes to protect healthy cells and inhibit cancer cells. Tests on mice with fish oils showed a reduction in spread of cancer tumours by 60 per cent. In this test omega 3 stopped the production of prostaglandins – hormone like substances that encourage cancer and poor cell division. Omega 3 oils replace and balance out omega 6 and other oils (notably saturated fats and cooking oils, somewhat typically, used in fast foods).

Walnut oil, olive oil, flaxseed oil and macadamia nut oil all contain omega 3 fatty acids but these are the short chain version and seem to be neutral in the body. As explained before, you should avoid taking too much cod liver oil as a supplement because of the possible overload on the body of vitamin A. 1,000 mgs once per day is the upper limit and even then you should have rest periods.

However, if you had to take three supplements to beat cancer and generally improve your health, they should be fish oils, fish oils and fish oils.

(iv) Glutathione

Glutathione is a very powerful antioxidant that helps neutralise rancid fats. It is a naturally occurring amino acid but the body can make it as well. Studies show clearly that, in older people those with the highest blood levels overcome illness quickest.

Glutathione is produced in all cells of the body, specifically to break down dangerous toxins and free radicals. It works in the gut, in the blood stream and in the cells. Its particular strength is with peroxides, the precursors of free radicals, and also with bad fats.

Brussel sprouts, cabbage, cauliflower and broccoli are the usual recommended providers but top of the list are avocado, asparagus, watermelon, grapefruit, boiled potatoes, strawberries, raw tomatoes, oranges, and orange juice.

You can take 100 mgs of glutathione with your meal. Also taking glutamine, an amino acid supplement, pumps up glutathione in the body and boosts the immune system. It can be taken as two teaspoons of glutamine powder (8,000 mgs) daily dissolved in water. Two to three times that volume may be needed if you are ill.

(v) Cysteine and cystine

Cystine is the stable form of a sulphur-based amino acid called cysteine. The body converts between the two. By taking the supplement L-cystine with vitamin C in a 1:3 ratio with food you can add further protection against free radical damage – particularly that from smoking, drinking and X-ray radiation. It also works to detoxify, and counter balance the carcinogenic factor homo-cysteine.

(vi) Shark cartilage

'Sharks don't get cancer', so the story goes. Sharks have no bones, only flexible cartilage. By taking this cartilage and pummelling it carefully, so that it breaks down without disrupting the active protein chains, treatments have been prepared from the resulting powder. As with soya isoflavones and garlic, the action of the protein is claimed to prevent or reduce the growth of cancers. It does this by restricting the blood supply to the cancer, called angeniosis (remember a tumour over 1cm needs its own blood supply). However after positive TV documentaries in the USA, many firms rushed out capsules. Critics claim that, even if these contained the right purified active ingredient, cancer sufferers would need to take almost a whole bottle per day.

It is however used by some clinics in its correct and pure form and apparently does have a positive effect.

(vii) Acidophilus

Lactobacillus acidophilus is a source of friendly intestinal bacteria. The friendly bacteria in the gut weigh in total about 1.5 kilos, and they are the first line of defence in the immune system. Antibiotics and even chlorine from tap water destroy friendly natives in the intestine, allowing an overgrowth of fungus to occur.

Lactose, pectin and vitamin C aid the growth of 'friendlies' (lactose is, however, a milk sugar). Acidophilus unfortunately can die off in just three days if your body is unbalanced or stressed, so topping up the bacteria on a regular basis is an insurance policy, especially since if the yeast fungus takes over it leaches vitamins, particularly B vitamins, and minerals from the system.

There is some indication that acidophilus, in standard pill form, may be destroyed by the pH in the stomach, thus preventing it from reaching the intestines. Slow release pills are apparently the answer to this problem.

If it is possible that you are susceptible to this type of yeast infection, you should avoid eating live bakers yeast and B complex vitamins with yeast.

There is some evidence that small pieces of the cell walls of friendly bacteria can pass through the lining of the intestine into the blood system. In tests, these bacteria wall pieces kill cancer cells.

(viii) Red wine

Red grapes, particularly cabernet grapes, contain high concentrations of catechins in their skins. Catechins block tumours and oxidative free radicals and inhibit bacteria and viruses. One glass of cabernet sauvignon twice a week would be helpful.

(ix) Eating less calories than you need

You may have read about the rats that were fed 40 per cent less food and lived to the equivalent of 140 years of age. There are huge benefits in calorie restriction for humans too:

- Eating too much bombards your cells with free radicals. The less calories you consume, the less energy is made in the power stations in your cells, so the less waste toxins and free radicals you produce. An excess of free radicals affects the balance of your various hormones and reduces communication between them.
- Calorie restriction causes an increase in protective enzymes and, if it occurs over a lengthy and continuous period, stimulates the production of melatonin and human growth hormone both of which neutralise free radicals.
- Calorie restriction reduces the likelihood of excess insulin production and less insulin means less bad eicosanoids. It also reduces excess blood glucose, known to damage the hypothalamus, the control centre for all hormones.

So it's not just the rats that benefit. In the war the Germans took away much of the Norwegians' food, leaving them on a calorie restricted diet with a high fish content. During those five years the heart attack rate fell significantly.

There is further evidence that eating less reduces the cancer risk in humans. The Okinawans have a calorie-restricted diet. They eat three times more vegetables and twice as much fish as the average Japanese but far less rice, animal protein, and fat resulting in a healthier diet but also a consumption of about 20–40 per cent less calories.

Their cancer rate is 60 per cent less.

106

(x) Medicinal mushrooms and glycoproteins

Over the last two decades Nobel prizes in physiology and medicine have gone to people looking at, for example, how the brain communicates with cells or how cells themselves communicate. When the nuclear DNA wants to direct your body to make green eyes or five toes it makes a protein message. But it has to tag this message with a post-code so that it ends up in the right destination.

In 1999 Dr Gunter Blobel won the Nobel prize for showing how the protein messages have this post-code in them, how they pass across protein cell walls, and how errors in this system can be linked to cancer, aids, the herpes virus and heredity diseases.

Some of this work had led already to drugs being produced, and one alone Arithroprotein, is a $2 bn business in the USA.

Certain saccharides (special protein/sugar like compounds) seem to have a role in helping this message system work effectively.

Sources for these saccharides include Japanese and Chinese mushrooms, onions, garlic, shellfish, bovine cartilage, breast milk, pectins (apples and citrus fruit eaten whole), aloe vera and arabinogalactin (in corn, leeks, radishes, peas, red wine, coconut, curcumin, rice, psyllium, echinacea, tomatoes, carrots and the bark of certain trees).

Shitake, maitake, reishi and cordycep mushrooms have been shown to have anti-cancer properties. Medicinal mushrooms contain bio-available beta glucan polysaccharide which is a proven anti-mutagen (ie stops the formation of the first rogue); it increases apoptosis and reduces skin cancer in mice. The use of mushroom nutrition is standard practice in many orthodox Japanese cancer treatments.

In a recent paper from Strathclyde University medicinal mushrooms also improved immune system strength, reduced side effects of both radio and chemotherapy, improved the quality of life amongst long-term cancer patients and improved survival rates.

A survey in one region of Japan, and covered in November

2002 by Cancer Research UK, showed that the mushroom pickers had 66 per cent less cancer than the surrounding population. 'Scrumping' has its benefits.

Q22. Learn to eat properly!

Ask any woman who has bad pre-menstrual pains how rapidly they are eased by evening primrose oil; or over-eat beetroot or asparagus and see how quickly your urine is affected. What you eat and drink affects your body quite rapidly, so it is wise to eat properly. Here are a few tips:

- If vegetables are eaten raw at the start of a meal (eg crudités, or raw vegetables with some dips), up to 40 per cent more vitamins and minerals are absorbed.
- Consumption of water before, during or at the end of the meal should be avoided. Excess water merely dilutes the digestive enzymes and prevents them from working fully. Drink copious amounts of water but at least one and a half hours from a meal.
- Eat slowly and focus on the food. Reading, working or watching TV can cause a whole range of emotions and stress to alter your hormone balance and prevent the perfect uptake of vitamins and minerals.
- Chew thoroughly. This releases an enzyme in the saliva called ptyalin which is crucial to the proper digestion of carbohydrates. Try and eat four to six small meals per day to maintain your blood sugar levels and put less strain on your digestive tract and endocrine system.
- Do not eat carbohydrate and protein at the same time. In the wild, our natural environment saw us find tubers and eat them, or gorge at a fruit tree, or capture an animal. We didn't take them all back to the cave and eat them on the same plate! Your digestive system is not designed for this total simultaneous consumption.

The carbohydrate and ptyalin mixture passes to the stomach where it needs an alkaline environment for maximum efficiency. Carbohydrate on its own clears the stomach in about one hour.

Protein on the other hand passes to the stomach where it meets its digestive enzyme pepsin and this requires an acid environment. Protein on its own can be digested in about one and a half hours.

But mix the two and the stomach doesn't know whether to be

alkaline or acid, with the result that the food is improperly digested and takes up to eight hours to pass through. This results in inefficiency throughout the intestinal system.

- Fruits should always be consumed first, at the start of the meal and on an empty stomach. Otherwise they can sit on top of a meal and ferment, causing toxins to be produced. People on anti-yeast diets need to avoid this complication as the fermentation aids the growth of yeasts.
- Vegetables, pulses, and oats, for example, contain soluble fibre. This is essential to the alimentary canal where it dissolves, transports, and helps excrete toxins and excess hormones. Rice should be eaten at least once a day (preferably organic whole and brown), as it is particularly good at cleaning your system.
- Eat fresh vegetables, fresh herbs, and fresh fruit. And try to eat them as close to the raw state as possible. Raw or steamed vegetables retain their nourishment values best, whilst boiling tends to reduce vitamin and mineral levels. But you don't just get vitamins and minerals from vegetables. When you pick broccoli it has an energy field, an aura. Despite steaming, broccoli retains most of this energy and the aura can still be seen in special photographs. If you microwave broccoli, all the energy and aura is lost. Little work has been done on this subject but quite possibly our absorption of the energy of our foodstuffs is as important as the vitamin and mineral content.
- Restrict meat and fish to four times per week. Have vegetarian days. Pulses are an excellent protein source for these non-meat days. Why have non-meat days? I have already talked about animal fats. In a research study on women in northern Italy commissioned by New York University, two similar groups of women were studied, both of which ate lots of carbohydrate and olive oil, but the group consuming meat and dairy had three times the cancer risk.
- If a woman cuts her fat intake in half, her oestrogen level will fall 20 per cent or more.
- Because fat is a good solvent, animal fat actually accumulates toxins the animal ate or produced. Meat and fish also bring their hormones into your body.

- Cooking meat produces carcinogens. The most dangerous is the production of nitrosamines from meat being burnt, or from the smoke of the coals or wood, on barbecues. Even when animal proteins are heated they produce heterocyclic amines and grilled chicken is 15 times worse than beef! (Sinha, Rothman, Brown (1995) *Cancer Research*).
- The World Health Organisation (WHO) has recently confirmed that acrylamides cause cancer. In January 2002, acrylamides were found by Swedish researchers in chips, crisps, breakfast cereals, crispbreads, biscuits, and other foods cooked (usually baked) at very high temperatures.
- Fried food in general is bad for you. Fried meat is linked to a higher risk of hormone related cancers in women, and men who eat fried food regularly have a three times higher risk than people who eat it in moderation.
- Stomach cancer is linked with smoked, pickled, salted or dried foods, where sodium nitrite is used as a preserving agent.
- Pickled foods, alcohol and tobacco increase cancer risk in the oesophagus. Meat, alcohol and coffee are turning the previously low rates of pancreatic cancer in Japan into Western numbers.

Quite simply we all need to get back to basics. Eating properly requires effort and time. Don't bring certain foods into the house in the first place; modify your cooking and eating habits and start all your planning with fruit and vegetables.

Q23. Which natural foods offer the best sources of the important vitamins and minerals?

If the UK Government's recommendation is that you should eat five helpings of fresh fruit and vegetables a day, what is a helping? If someone has five boiled potatoes, is that the Government's view of providing daily health?

Meanwhile, the French Government wants its population to eat 10 portions. Who is right and where is the justification for this?

First the Government has to be clear on its recommendations and make them less woolly and more relevant to the population. Then a total education programme needs to be started, in schools and through advertising and PR, which encourages children and their parents to understand what is really being recommended and why.

But in the short term, where do you go to provide a good diet with the required levels of, say antioxidants? Well, often it is not the fruit and veg. Here is a simple guide to some of the best natural sources of each vitamin or mineral in the fight against cancer:

Vitamin E

2 tablespoons of sunflower seeds	11 mgs
1 tablespoon sunflower oil	6 mgs
20 almonds	8 mgs
1 tablespoon of soya oil	3 mgs
1 tablespoon of wheatgerm	3 mgs

You can see from this that it is hard to get near the ideal level of 400 IU of vitamin E naturally per day (400 IU = 268 mgs) without taking vitamin supplements. Throw sunflower seeds on salads, have a bowl of pumpkin, sunflower and sesame seeds to nibble rather than crisps or peanuts.

Vitamin C

1 large red pepper	224 mgs
100 gms raw broccoli	90 mgs
150 gms papaya	90 mgs
1 large orange	65 mgs

Surprisingly then the top vitamin C producer is not an orange! Your morning glass of orange juice only gives you about 10 mgs and is usually pasteurised and full of sugar unless you have squeezed it yourself. So it's chopped red pepper with everything and broccoli as raw as possible (but wash it well).

Beta-carotene

1 cup carrot juice	24.2 mgs
1 medium sweet potato	10.0 mgs
5 dried apricots	6.2 mgs
1 cup red cherries	6.2 mgs
½ cup cooked spinach	5.7 mgs
1 cup tomato juice	2.2 mgs

Beta-carotene is plentiful in nature in colourful foods and green vegetables. Red and yellow peppers, tomatoes and kale are others.

Lycopene

1 standard tin of tomato soup	65 mgs
1 tin of vegetable juice	23 mgs
5 tablespoons of tomato paste	22 mgs
5 tablespoons of tomato ketchup	12 mgs

So you need to look little further than tomatoes. The next best are watermelons. Studies show men who eat seven servings a week of tomatoes and tomato products reduce their prostate risk by 40 per cent. Cooked tomatoes are best as they release their lycopene more easily to your digestive system.

Zinc

6 oysters	55 mgs
Medium serving of steak	8 mgs

| 4 tablespoons of sunflower seeds | 6 mgs |
| Serving of All Bran | 4 mgs |

Well it's oysters every day now! Zinc is ubiquitous and you are only trying to get to 15–25 mgs per day.

Selenium

4 cracked brazil nuts in shells	150 mcgs
4 slices of wholemeal bread	60 mcgs
2 tablespoons sunflower seeds	15 mcgs
1 egg	15 mcgs
1 skinless chicken breast	10 mcgs

Try to avoid brazil nuts (or any nuts) in cellophane wrappers as depending upon their shelf time they may be rancid. Crack them yourself.

Omega 3 fatty acids

Salmon	1.0 mgs per gm
Herring	1.0 mgs per gm
Mackerel	0.9 mgs per gm

As we covered with eicosanoids, fish oils provide omega 3 in a most concentrated form. Mackerel wins in terms of overall health because it has least total fat.

Calcium

| 100 gms tinned sardines | 460 mgs |
| 100 gms almonds | 250 mgs |

By comparison a glass of skimmed milk gives only 120 mgs and 150 gm low fat yoghurt gives 190 mgs.

Just from this brief study you can see how easy it is to reach your targets, and that is without the five helpings of fruit and vegetables a day, although they do play a crucial role with the fibre you need. It is also important to restrict the amount of fruit within this mix to two to three pieces a day as not all leave alkaline ash in the body, as we saw earlier.

Q24. Are there any specific diets that could be useful?

Before we get into specific diets, there are a couple of possible additions to the anti-cancer armoury that are worth knowing.

(a) The juice fast

Dr Otto Buchinger Jr is considered by many to be the leading expert in this area and he calls juice fasts, 'the royal road to healing'. Using a good juicer and organically grown produce, you first soak the fruit and vegetables in a big bowl of water containing 1 capful of peroxide to remove bacteria, chemical residues and parasites.

Raw juices like carrot, beetroot, celery, cabbage, apple, and watercress can be surprisingly tasty. Add a little ginger to help the taste if you wish. They are extremely cleansing, easy to digest, and packed full of vitamins, minerals and enzymes.

The detoxification process, which should be used for three to seven days, may result at first in some side effects like headaches, bad breath, tiredness, dizziness and even memory loss but health comes back with a vengeance.

The fast can be helped by:

- Liver cleansers like milk-thistle and other herbs;
- Colon cleansers like psyllium, alfalfa, goldenseal, and slippery elm.
- Aloe vera which helps kill bacteria, viruses, yeasts and helps to heal the damage from radiation and chemotherapy.
- Bromelain and papain, both of which are digestive enzymes that hit foreign substances including cancer cells.

You may also use blood cleansers like kelp, chlorella (which in particular binds heavy metals), and Essiac, which also helps to clean the liver and gallbladder and expel toxins in the gut. The latter is an excellent all round agent. Question 15 provides details on more general detoxing.

Immune system boosters can be taken at the same time. For example, echinacea which also cleans the blood and lymph systems, cat's claw and astralagus. (See Question 20)

(b) The coffee enema

You must be joking! No seriously, it has a very big fan club amongst alternative health doctors and practitioners. Enemas, like colonic irrigation, remove the toxins from the colon. The presence of organic coffee with caffeine stimulates the liver to cleanse itself (conversely actually drinking coffee poisons the whole system with caffeine) and opens up the bile ducts into the intestine. Stomach massage and castor oil also help clear out the toxins and prevent them being re-absorbed. The main draw back is that, with some cancer treatments, four enemas are recommended per day, each in all taking about 60–90 minutes. Coffee enemas are used by a lot of major cancer clinics.

Diets

The principle of, 'You are what you eat' stems from naturopathy and the belief that we are at one with our surroundings. The opposite of health is illness. There is only one state of health and all illness is one; it is just represented in a number of forms. If cancer is brought on by poor nourishment, then good nourishment is the way to beat it.

(i) The macrobiotic diet

In Greek 'macro' means great, and 'biotic' means concerning life. Macrobiotics, or the greater view of life, is based on the ancient Chinese understanding of yin and yang in the universe and is not confined to diet at all. The Chinese believe that everything in the universe can be divided into these two categories (think mother or father aspect), although it is fluid and one form can change into the other.

Between 1896 and 1907 Sagen Ishizuka, a Japanese army doctor developed a theory of nutrition. In it he combined both the Western medical thinking with ancient Oriental thinking. His basic tenet was that the food we eat not only sustains life but underpins our health and happiness.

During this period of time Japan was being heavily Westernised and he argued strongly against it, recommending re-adoption of the traditional Japanese diet, ie whole, unrefined foods with little or no milk or animal food. He set up a clinic and treated hundreds of patients with a traditional diet based on brown rice and a variety of land and sea vegetables. Such was his success that he became known as the 'Anti-Doctor'.

His five principles were:
1. Foods are the foundation of health and happiness
2. Sodium and potassium are opposites in food, and control its yin and yang character.
3. Grain is properly the staple food of man
4. Food should be unrefined, whole, and natural
5. Food should be grown locally and in season

Macrobiotic diets also require that foods are eaten as near the natural state as possible and cooking is almost an art form.

The use of a macrobiotic diet requires that there is an understanding of the patient's yin and yang state and that foods are then provided to correct any imbalance. The detail of their use for say the cancer patient, is beyond the scope of this book. You should telephone your local centre, contact the Macrobiotic Association and/or go to the website for a better understanding of how a macrobiotic diet might fit your personal needs. A fundamental part of macrobiotics is that everyone of us is different and one man's grain is another man's poison. So you must check it out thoroughly before you act on any advice. But the evidence is clear. A basic Japanese diet is much, much better for your health than a Western diet.

(ii) The Bristol Cancer Centre diet

This has been prepared for cancer sufferers by the Bristol Cancer Help Centre. It is not a diet therapy in its own right but guidelines and recommendations for a diet in support of other cancer treatments.

The guidelines suggest:
- consuming a large variety of fresh vegetables and fruits, especially raw
- increasing the range of grains you eat, especially wholegrain, to include quinoa, brown rice, barley and millet
- including beans and lentils at least three times per week and avoiding added bran

117

- eating nuts and seeds (sesame, sunflower, poppy, pumpkin).
- only using cold pressed plant oils for cooking and dressings (eg olive oil, sunflower oil)
- using freshly made organic fruit and vegetable juices where possible
- drinking 2 litres of filtered or bottled water per day.

Avoiding:

- red meat (beef, lamb or pork)
- saturated fat (milk, cream, cheese, yoghurt) – substituting soya
- smoked and salt cured foods
- refined sugar (use honey if necessary)
- processed and refined foods, which have preservatives.
- salt and sugar
- caffeine in coffee, tea, chocolate, and fizzy drinks
- excess alcohol
- sweet fizzy drinks.

The Bristol Cancer Centre also has courses covering meditation, visualisation and diet. It embraces holistic doctors, healers, nutritional therapists and counsellors.

Q25. What about cancer clinics?

This is a vast subject, since there are many clinics offering a variety of alternative and complementary treatments in a number of countries.

Because some doctors, despite holding very open-minded views on different potential ways of treating cancer, have used treatments like B-17, some of their clinics have been forced outside the system in the USA. This has allowed mainstream critics to dub them 'quacks', when some of their treatments may have merit. The resulting 'them and us' stance blocks proper clinical trials taking place, with the result that there is no firm evidence to support their work and their claims. This does all cancer patients a disservice.

One branch of the alternative/complementary clinics has developed its beliefs around the pancreas.

In 1911 a Scottish anatomist, **John Beard**, expounded theories about foetal cells and how, although they are rapidly dividing at first, this rate of division is switched to a more normal growth rate by an unknown controlling mechanism. Later in life new cells form in, for example, your eyes or your lungs from these original 'stem cells' but then something differentiates between the various types of cell. The work was developed further by **Dr William Kelley** in America. The theory was constructed that the controlling force was somehow provided by the pancreas. When cancer cells form they generate with the characteristics of foetal cells or stem cells, and are not differentiated. So lung cancer cells don't look like lung cells and are rapidly dividing.

Kelley believed everyone of us has their own personal metabolic code. His aim was to find this unique metabolism and stimulate it.

Kelley theorised that the formation of cancer was clear. **Excess female hormones were responsibile for changing a stem cell into a trophoblast cell.** In simple English, this means that cancer is the growth of normal tissue, but at the wrong time and in the wrong place. It progresses because of a lack of cancer digesting enzymes in the body and Kelley believed the pancreas, through its enzymes, was the primary cancer fighter in the body. So his solution was to get pancreatic enzymes to the cancer site and inhibit the growth, but control the rate of attack, or toxins would flood the body and cause problems elsewhere.

Kelley's treatment was divided into five parts:

1. **Nutritional therapy** – to break down the cancer cells; megavitamins, minerals, high dose vitamin C, bioflavenoids, coenzymes, raw almonds, amino acids and raw beef formula with pancreatic enzymes.

2. **Detoxification** – to cleanse the dead cells and toxins from the body; laxative purges, Epsom salts, fasts, lemon juice, coffee enemas (for anything from three weeks to 12 months)

3. **Diet** – to rebalance the body, the cellular metabolism and the immune system; at the outset he advocated a strict vegetarian diet, but modified this as he identified different individual types. In all he ended up with 10 different diet types and 95 variations. All diets forbade processed foods, pesticide residues, refined foods, peanuts, milk etc. They did allow almonds, low protein grains, nuts, organic raw fruits and vegetables.

4. **Neurological stimulation** – to allow free flow of body energy, especially to cancer site; for example, using osteopaths, chiropractors or physiotherapists. (A modern equivalent might be the use of a cranial osteopath to manipulate not just the skeletal structure but the free-flow of body energy.)

5. **Spiritual** – to lift the spirits, and call upon the universal good; Kelley urged patients to trust in God, to read The Bible and to pray.

Kelley monitored a patient's progress using his own Kelley Malignancy System. Over a 20 year period he reputedly treated 455 patients with 26 different cancers and claimed excellent results.

Even Ernst Krebs (of B-17 fame) followed this view of the pancreas.

Dr Nicholas Gonzales is a New York immunologist who has a clinic with Dr Linda Isaacs.

They have based their cancer treatment on Kelley's work, which they have refined and added to.

Gonzalez treatment dispenses with the neurological and spiritual elements. As with Kelley, Gonzalez believes cancer can be eliminated by the patient's own body, if the intestines, liver, kidneys, lungs and blood are all detoxified and the body's acid/alkaline pH and mineral and enzyme strengths are all in balance.

He uses his own system of hair analysis for monitoring progress.

Dr Gonzalez himself has been working on cancers since 1981. The results of his first clinical trial were published in June 1999, and his work on pancreatic cancer is currently being evaluated in a large-scale study. The clinic treats all cancers, although it is best known for pancreatic cancers, and also covers a number of other illnesses from chronic fatigue to multiple sclerosis.

The Gonzalez regime has just three basic units each modified for the particular individual being treated.

1. **Detoxification** – involves procedures such as coffee enemas (twice per day) to clean, purify and re-energise the liver. This in turn clears toxins out and improves the efficiency of the whole system.

2. **Diet** – individually designed diets using organic foods are used. Refined foods (sugar, flour, grains) are avoided, as are all processed and synthetic foods. Whilst some patients are on vegan diets using high levels of raw foods, others might be allowed two to three helpings of red meat.

3. **Supplements** – large doses of vitamins and minerals are used, including trace elements. Plus concentrates from glands and anti-oxidants and pancreatic enzymes, which whilst working as digestive aids, are also believed to represent the body's main cancer defence system.

In fact, Gonzalez believes that pancreatic enzymes actually liquefy tumours. It is not unusual for a patient to take 150–180 supplements along with 45 gms of pancreatic enzymes spread throughout the day.

He has produced studies of 50 patients, showing that all are alive 10 years later.

The **Gerson Therapy** is based around the hourly consumption of freshly prepared organic juices, which not only detox, but keep up high vitamin and particularly mineral levels in the body re-establishing a healthy metabolism. It was developed by Dr Max Gerson who had a number of successful clinics. Dr Albert Schweitzer called him, 'one of medicine's most eminent geniuses'. Gerson died in 1959 so there is no doubt he was ahead of his time in suggesting certain causes of cancer and in his belief that you had to attack the cause not the symptoms.

This treatment is a whole body treatment incorporating the principles of detoxification of the wastes and toxins that interfere with healing and normal metabolism, and an intensive nutritional programme to flood the body with healing nutrients. Thirteen fresh organic juices are consumed everyday and enemas, including the coffee enema, are used to detox. The juices are made from over 20 pounds of organically grown nuts and vegetables daily; one glass, 13 times. Some organic vegetables and fruits are consumed whole. The metabolism is also stimulated by the addition of thyroid, potassium and other supplements.

The therapy has its critics. Gerson's view that a natural diet would restore the body's resistance and healing power lost through years of artificial nutrition meant he openly criticised a lot of modern foods and these are banned from the diet, for example, dairy, wheat, caffeine, animal fat, excess protein, and sodium.

The Gerson Institute is in San Diego, but Californian law does not permit them to treat patients there. They now have a clinic in Mexico and a centre in Liverpool, England. Qualified support groups exist on a more local basis.

The Gerson therapy can even be adopted at home, although proper medical supervision is recommended.

Dr Lawrence Plaskett in the UK is a long time admirer of the pioneering work of Gerson in the 1940s and 1950s. Dr Plaskett currently holds the vice-chair of the Nutritional Therapy Council in the UK.

Plaskett had long offered nutritional treatment in his practice and decided to design a new therapy based on a common medical philosophy with Gerson, but incorporating many of the newer nutritional discoveries and biochemical advances. Using his nutritional expertise and incorporating a lengthy and detailed study of the research literature available covering anti-carcinogenic and anti-tumour nutrients, foods and nutriceuticals, Plaskett developed a completely separate therapy.

The therapy consists of a very specific diet, nutritional supplement programme, herbs, juices, coffee enemas and even some complex naturopathic remedies. It embodies variations that take into account the differing needs of patients with cancers of different types.

Dr Plaskett now has a college which trains practitioners in nutritional medicine and he no longer treats patients these days. Instead, he has passed his therapy on to the National Cancer Therapy Trust (NCTT) for practical application in the UK. There are over 70 fully qualified practitioners working with the Trust throughout the UK, and since 1997 those patients who have been able to take the therapy fully and consistently have shown remarkable results.

Dr Patrick Kingsley works near Leicester in England. He treats a whole spectrum of patients, some of whom have cancer. These patients may or may not have had orthodox medical treatment first.

An open-minded gentleman, Dr Kingsley has no one treatment. He believes in identifying the cause of the cancer and what might be sustaining it and then treating that cancer with the appropriate mix of diet and therapy. He encourages positive thinking and might use a wide variety of treatments from B-17 to digestive enzymes.

One possible treatment, for example, is intravenous use of megadose vitamin C and hydrogen peroxide. The theory runs that the peroxide oxygen attacks the fastest growing cells in the body and cancer cells are killed by oxygen, whilst the vitamin C protects the normal cells from danger.

His diet recommends avoiding tea, coffee, milk and all dairy, wheat and yeasts, refined carbohydrates, sugars and junk food. He advises consumption of soya products, fresh organic fruits and vegetables (especially cruciferous eg broccoli, cabbage) and

123

10 gms of Ester-C per day (Ester-C is the non-acid version of vitamin C and supposedly kinder on the stomach) with large amounts of antioxidant vitamins plus 7–10 gms of echinacea. He also uses coffee enemas.

One report suggested he had a two-third success rate.

The Dove Clinic in the UK provides an integrated approach to cancer treatment. Its doctors are conventionally medically trained, but also have experience and qualifications in a range of complementary disciplines. Led by **Dr Julian Kenyon**, they have an extremely open minded and wide approach to cancer treatment ranging from immune system testing to nutritional medicine. Treatments include activated oxygen, vitamin C megadoses, immune therapy and cancer vaccines through to photodynamic therapy. This latter and recent development uses algae to impregnate cells. After a couple of days, the algae only remains in the cancerous cells and these can be killed by exposing them to light. Although in its early stages, results have been impressive.

It is quite clear that the treatment of cancer cannot be confined to the 'holy trinity' of orthodox medicine, namely surgery, radiotherapy and chemotherapy. All of these can work, but then so can a number of other treatments.

The most important factors in the treatment of cancer are having an open mind, and then providing some serious evidence of effectiveness. Sadly the above clinics seem to have to work doubly hard to prove themselves.

Q26. Can screening help beat cancer?

All the best advice is that the earlier you discover a cancer the greater your odds are of beating it. Screening can play an important part in this process. Basically screening can be simplified under three headings.

(i) Tried and trusted methods?

Palpation (looking for a lump with your fingers)

Women over 30 should examine their **breasts** at least every month. In the USA if you have ever had radiation treatment on the chest region, it is recommended that start self-screening much earlier. The self-test should be performed seven to ten days after the start of the menstrual period, since the texture and density of the breast tissue will change during the monthly cycle. Women who are post-menopausal should choose the same day every month.

Firstly conduct a visual examination studying the size, dimpling, and shape of each breast including the nipple. Then gently feel your breasts using the pads of your three longest fingers looking for lumps, bumps and changes. A fuller description can be obtained from the breast cancer charity (see page 230 for contact details).

Mammography

Years of usage of the mammogram, especially in the USA, has created a popular belief in its importance. And during the 70s and 80s as mammograms came into widespread use, coupled with early detection and a greater consciousness of breast cancer, breast cancer deaths fell by 30 per cent.

Mammograms provide a detailed image of the breast tissue. If the tissue is soft, detection of an unusual lump is relatively easy, but becomes harder the more 'lumpy' the breast tissue. The problem is that women most at risk of breast cancer are far more likely to have dense breast tissue, making emerging small tumours very hard to spot.

Doctors recommend women over 40 should have the test annually as early detection provides better rates of cure and can offer the choice of a lumpectomy rather than a full mastectomy. However, each mammogram delivers a high dose of radiation – up to 1,000 times that of a normal X-ray – and there is much debate as to whether the mammograms themselves do more harm than good.

A two-year study in Denmark, originally published in the Lancet and updated in October 2001 suggests that a number of flaws in the mammography process makes the test 'virtually useless'. This has caused controversy and even anger amongst the medical profession.

Dr Kelly McMasters, a surgical oncologist at the University of Louisville is quite clear that the current technology is still showing results and is a lot better than examining yourself. 'The problem with palpation is that when a tumour is big enough to feel it's often spread already to the lymph nodes. This makes it more likely to be fatal'.

The jury is out, and women should make absolutely sure they understand all the risks, and whether they will feel confident in the results.

Testicular self-examination
It is not hard to examine the testes. Testicular cancer is most common in the 15-40 age group. The test should be carried out monthly after a warm shower, by rolling the each testicle slowly and gently between the thumb and fingers. Any small lump or hard object should be examined by a doctor. Other signs to watch for are dull aches in the testicle, groin or abdomen. This is a highly curable disease especially if caught early.

Sigmoidoscopy
A sigmoidoscope is a narrow tube with a light at the end. Inserted in the rectum it can find polyps and tumours in the lower colon. By contrast a colonoscopy is a longer tube and looks further in to the colon. A newer system called flexible sigmoidoscopy, aims to detect precancerous growths using a miniature camera inserted into the bowel.

The UK Health Minister announced at a national cancer conference that he is intending to introduce a national bowel cancer screening programme for everybody over the age of 50, and is awaiting final results from a Cancer Research UK study.

Two approaches to screening are under consideration, one of which involves testing faeces for early signs of cancer, while the other uses sigmoidoscopy to detect the pre-cancerous growths.

Pap smear

Created by Dr Papaniculaou in the 1940s it has been a major contributor to the lowered rates of **cervical cancer** since that time. The test can detect both pre-cancerous and cancerous cells in the cervix.

The test involves inserting a speculum into the vagina so the cervix can be clearly seen. Sample cells are then taken from the outer part of the cervix using a spatula and using a brush from the inner part. A pelvic examination is also conducted at the same time. An annual smear is recommended after the commencement of sexual activity.

Tumour markers

A number of factors are to be found in the blood each indicating the presence of a cancer. Measuring their presence and level can be helpful not just to indicate the cancer but to monitor the effectiveness of treatments.

PSA test

If you are 50 years or over and living in the West there is a very good chance you will have an enlarged non-malignant **prostate** (termed benign prostatic hyperplasia). This carries with it certain symptoms, which are virtually identical to those of prostate cancer.

The UK charity, The Prostate Cancer Charity, defines them as:

- Difficulty or pain when passing urine
- The need to pass urine more often
- Broken sleep due to the need to pass urine
- Waiting for long periods before the urine flows
- The feeling that the bladder has not completely emptied.

With prostate cancer you may also suffer from blood in the urine, and/or lower back pain and/or dribbling. But be aware that many of the above symptoms can be caused by other factors eg bacterial infection.

Your doctor can simply feel if you have an enlarged prostate (a digital rectal examination). If he finds such an enlargement he will probably send you for a PSA test (prostate-specific antigen). This measures a specific protein in a man's blood, the level of which was thought to correlate with prostate cancer.

However, this test has been found to be flawed. In one research study, factors found in the blood from high dairy consumption, vigorous exercise, or riding a bicycle in the previous 24 hours increased PSA levels.

Indeed, the test does not seem to fully distinguish between enlarged malignant prostates and non-malignant ones, and one USA report concluded that as many as two thirds of those testing positive, probably are not!

CA125
CA125 levels can be used to detect ovarian cancer at an early stage. However although a number of other cancers can increase the level of CA125, so too can a number of benign conditions like endometriosis, fibroids and even pregnancy. For this reason the test is seen as flawed.

Pyruvate kinase
The majority of solid tumour cancers over-express this enzyme and this can aid detection.

Others
There are several current tests to ascertain whether a cancer is present. No one is particularly decisive but together they can give a reasonably accurate picture of events:

Interleukin and Interferon: can both show immune response levels

CA15-3 : breast cancer

CA19-9 : oesophageal, bile duct and pancreas

CEA   : oesophageal, lung, bile, colon, pancreas and bladder.
However as before, no one of these is perfect and a complex picture has to be studied.

Now scientists from the Federal Drug Agency (FDA) and

National Cancer Institute (NCI) in the USA have reported on another as yet unnamed protein test taking just 30 minutes and using a small sample of patient's blood. Although the authors caution that more work is needed to understand the sensitivity of the test, the initial tests identified 50 out of 50 cancer, and 63 out of 66 non-cancer samples.

There is no doubt accurate protein tests could be of significant benefit. For example, currently more than 80 per cent of ovarian cancer patients are diagnosed at a late clinical stage and have a less than 20 per cent chance of five-year survival. In contrast early diagnosis results in 95 per cent survival over the same period making the possibility of protein tests a truly exciting development.

For more information use: www.cancer.gov/newscenter.

(ii) Some examples of new methods being developed

The camera you swallow

The M2A is a camera the size of a vitamin pill and developed by the US firm Given Imaging. When swallowed this battery powered device generates 57,000 images as it passes through the stomach and through the intestine. To date it has been used at the Royal Hallamshire Hospital to discover the causes of intestinal bleeding, but its potential to study polyps, tumours and bowel cancer is enormous. At £300 a time it is the ultimate disposable camera!

Testicular scanner on trial

The world's largest trial to see if a new scanner can improve treatment for testicular cancer patients has been launched by Cancer Research UK.

Scientists funded by the charity will use a sophisticated Positron Emission Tomography (PET) scan to search for early signs of cancer spread in order to identify those at risk of relapse after surgery.

The PET scanner relies on differences in the way tumour cells and normal tissue metabolise glucose to hunt down the active tumour tissue.

New prostate tests

Scientists now believe they have a way to identify **prostate** cancers, which are aggressive and those that are not. To date measurement has always looked at the stage, or spread, of the cancer but there has been little evidence on the grade, or how rapidly the cancer is growing. The problem is that some men with small, yet rapidly growing cancers have not been spotted in time. Now scientists can test the tumours of newly diagnosed patients to discover how aggressive the cancer is. The test involves measuring the amount of an enzyme present in the blood. This enzyme is only produced by cancer cells.

A trial, reported in the scientific journal *Cancer* in September 2002, involved 105 prostate surgery samples. The test is probably applicable to **breast** and **colon** cancers as well.

(iii) Genetic testing

An example:

Women can now be screened for the presence of faulty BRCA1 and BRCA2 genes. Genes are little messages sitting on the ball of string which is your DNA. These are dubbed erroneously the 'breast cancer genes' as, in the 10 per cent of women who have these genes, breast cancer is a high risk. In fact BRCA1 is connected with the immune system and BRCA2 with DNA repair. Both genes have also been linked to a percentage of colon and prostate cancers whilst other, similar genes have been identified for colon and other cancer risks.

The hope is that drugs can be developed to switch off these genes, if their mechanism of cause can be accurately determined. For the time being women identified as having these genes are offered preventative mastectomies or the drug Tamoxifen. This drug has been shown to have benefits, but also it is itself classified as a carcinogen by the World Health Organisation, as it has definite cancer causing risks.

It is appropriate that women with these genes are not influenced by scare mongering, but do take sensible lifestyle precautions.

SECTION III

You are more than just
a machine

'Mind over matter'

Introduction

I walked out of my hotel in the middle of China early one cold December morning and saw a fascinating sight. About 80 Chinese, the youngest in their 60s, all fully clothed and complete with jackets and hats to brave the weather, were standing practising t'ai chi in rows in a dusty square. Slow movements as graceful as a thick coat would allow. No one broke sweat and certainly no one experienced 'the burn'.

As we went off to the medical centre on our two hour journey by bus, we saw perhaps just 50 cars or lorries but literally thousands of people of all ages on their bicycles.

At the medical centre the doctor looked at my eyes, tongue and ears. He told me I had a colon problem and gave me herbs. In London the same diagnosis had required three specialists, X-rays and a barium meal.

I was taken for a massage, offered acupuncture and shown how this was used in place of anaesthetic in operations. The doctor was in fact very open-minded and objective about Western medicine and claimed he would certainly use it if it offered better results.

China had a terrible infant mortality record in the past but this is improving rapidly. According to my Chinese doctor, remove infant mortality from the life expectancy figures and the Chinese would expect to live longer than Europeans or Americans. What will we do if one day those figures are clearly borne out in the West? Will our medical authorities be as open-minded or keen to learn?

133

Q27. How are we really doing on cancer prevention and cure?

Modern medicine undeniably has helped us to live longer, wiping out diseases and infections that used to kill. But its conquests are becoming less and less effective as the tide of illness mounts.

The average life expectancy of an American in 1900 was 48. By 1920 it was 57 and by 1990 any new baby could expect to live to 75. Great strides.

However, if you take out infant mortality from the figures and ask how long if you were 50 would you expect to live, in 1920, he or she could expect to live to 74; and by 1990 to 78. This 7–8 per cent improvement is no mean achievement but far less than many people would suppose across a 70 year period, considering all the money that has been poured into research, medicines, and the health services.

Since 1980 this age-adjusted life expectancy figure has hardly increased at all.

The five year survival rates for people with cancer in the USA improved by about 10 per cent between 1974 and 1990, going from 49 per cent to 54 per cent. However since 1990 this figure has remained virtually static.

Statistically, early detection has not increased cure rates and, with a couple of very notable exceptions (eg child leukaemia), a large number of current treatments do not seem to prolong over-all life. Perhaps this is because, whilst science advances, other factors like diet, stress and health risks are acting in the opposite direction. Perhaps the emphasis on the curative route the medical profession is taking is not the right approach.

Take cancer death ages and there is little difference over time. The average age of death from cancer has hardly changed in 15 years. Part of the reason for this is that more younger people are contracting it.

More people now contract cancer. In the USA in 2001 there were 1.3 million new cases of cancer and 550,000 deaths. These figures have increased by 60 per cent since 1950. New cases are estimated to exceed 1.6 million by 2005.

In a survey of industrialised nations (including USA, Europe, and Japan) non-smoking related cancers account for 78 per cent of this growth, with a growth in prostate cancer of 200 per cent, breast cancer of 64 per cent, and child cancers of 35 per cent. Although Japan has cancer rates considerably lower than in the West, breast cancer has risen by 100 per cent in the same period.

In the UK there were around 260,000 new cases of cancer in the year 2001. Mortality levels were:

Lung cancer	34,250
Large bowel cancer	16,000
Breast cancer	13,500
Prostate cancer	9,500
Stomach cancer	7,000
Oesophageal cancer	7,000

Also, one has to be careful of exactly how the figures are presented. One oncologist told me that breast cancer sufferers had an 85 per cent chance of surviving five years and published data claims that over 75 per cent of cases are successfully treated. However a simple piece of maths shows that last year there were 39,500 new cases in the UK. In the same year 13,500 women died from it, a figure of 35 per cent of the new cases, indicating a 65 per cent survival rate. Obviously some of these are outside the five year period but it portrays a truer figure for overall survival rates. There are only a few cancers that can be genuinely totally cured despite the billions of pounds spent and the quality of the people involved.

The current Genome Project work may have enormous potential though. Scientists have mapped your complete DNA 'string', showing which parts correspond to your eyes, ears and legs; and also showing little pieces of code that determine cancers in your body. Scientists are currently working on how to switch off these pieces of code. However, whether they will be able to 'play' with your genes without causing extra problems in the body remains to be seen.

Different countries spend vastly different amounts on cancer cure . For example, the spending in 2000 on cancer therapy drugs per capita was:-

USA	$10.86
Germany	$8.74
Italy	$5.33
UK	$1.33

Sadly against all this activity little focus is placed on **prevention**.

As we saw in Section I, the Western world's weight of money from government, charities and drug companies pouring into cancer cures is quite incredible. Without wishing to seem cynical, this is because of several factors, none of which has much to do with the health of the nation. Hardly a day passes without a story in the national press about trials of a new wonder drug. It's good copy and it shows that people are trying. Charities want more money to explore cancers and look for cures so they can show successes and results. Governments want to support a health service that has sick patients sitting in queues. Drug companies have a symbiotic relationship with doctors and Governments to do their best to supply the cures, notwithstanding the profits they will make.

The rising rates of cancer have come about slowly across a 50 year or more period and reversing this trend could be expected to take a similar period, even if it were possible. Since most company bosses, presidents and prime ministers don't last much more than 50 months this doesn't come too high on their agendas. And anyway, given the high levels of non-smoking related cancers and their diversity, how could you afford the structures necessary to monitor all possible toxins and their effects in areas such as household or cosmetic or toiletry products or industrial waste and nuclear power stations or food crops and water supplies, or magnetic fields from aerials and power lines? Even where quite good controls already exist, how would you start scientifically to monitor and improve the interaction of it all?

These are the challenges facing us all. Clearly every thinking person who cares about the world they are passing on to the next generation ought to be making their voice heard and the government, schools and the media all have a role to play, but then so does every parent in the Western world doing the cooking or buying the household products. Meanwhile all we can try to do is to create our own little micro-environments as best we can. We all need to understand the carcinogens that attack us and the lifestyle elements that destroy us. We can at least take some sensible steps in the areas open to our own control. And, if the worst happens and we succumb to cancer, we need to realise that there are diet, medical, lifestyle and complementary approaches outside our standard Western medical thinking that definitely can help us all.

As Lily Tomlin once said, '*We're all in this together.... On our own!*'

Q28. Is it possible that 'scientific cancer cures' are not addressing the real problem?

There is a celebrated doctor and health guru called Deepak Chopra who runs a clinic called the Chopra Centre for Well Being in La Jolla, California. He believes fervently that you can not only stop the ravages of ageing and disease but with effort and care you can actually reverse them.

He, like a lot of people who have studied Eastern medicine, believes that the mind, body and soul are inexorably linked. Poor thoughts in the mind or depression take their toll on bodily performance. This is not some cranky thinking but now well established medically.

Every cell in your body is made up of atoms, which in turn are merely particles spinning round other particles in electromagnetic fields largely composed of air. Everyday your body takes in new atoms and expels others so that you completely change all the cells, and all the atoms, in your body every few weeks. Why should it not be possible to kick out a cancer if you could work out what caused it and moreover what exactly was sustaining it? If your diet or lifestyle gave you the cancer originally, why would it not be possible to change them both and return your body to its original healthy state?

The body must be seen as far, far more than the sum of the mechanical parts, and ultimately it will be totally understood that every single one of us has within us the ability to heal and repair a damaged part.

We've all heard stories of love healing, or the power of positive thinking overcoming disease, or even the power of prayer. But then our body is a summation of all these atoms in their magnetic fields within one enormous magnetic field, the universe. Of course there could be an interaction between two beings, or between your mind and the atoms in your liver; or between your energetic being and the energy of the universe.

It is most certainly the case that modern medicine will not

succeed in increasing cancer cure rates unless it takes a broader perspective and realises that it has to treat the total patient, rather than merely the cancer.

Now you may consider all this alternative stuff is for cranks, so let's look at a few random facts about the total you, even if indeed they do seem a little strange sometimes.

- More of the world believes in and uses complementary medicine than uses modern Western medicine. A better name for alternative medicine would be traditional, natural healing. In fact at least twice as many people in the world use diet and natural healing as use modern medicine. In the UK, 40 per cent of all cancer patients have at least one form of complementary therapy (Macmillan).
- One American study stated that with certain cancers an individual was two to three times more likely to achieve a cure through diet and supplements than through radiotherapy and chemotherapy combined.
- Certain cancers are almost non-existent in China and south east Asia; is this despite their diets, or because of them? Take a Chinese person to New York and they are statistically just as likely to develop a cancer as the native New Yorker.
- Animals like bears and gorillas never get cancer in the wild. Keeping them in zoos with unnatural diets and stressful surroundings causes seven out of 10 to get cancer.
- Researchers have found that women who have three orgasms a week have higher levels of immunoglobin A and boost their immune systems by up to 30 per cent! Apparently every time women reach orgasm their bodies produce more T lymphocytes to better resist infection and fight cancer. Good sex also produces growth hormone and releases endorphins, so-called happy hormones that neutralise anxiety and stress hormones in the body. If that wasn't enough girls, in a study of women with breast cancer those who had regular orgasms recovered faster than those who didn't.

- Reiki, or hands on healing, has so powerful an effect on the chakras (spiritual centres in the body) that it cannot be used whilst someone is having radiotherapy or chemotherapy because its healing power reduces their effectiveness.
- Chinese doctors do not like to poison the immune system of their patients with anaesthetics. They operate using acupuncture leaving the patient with no after-effects at the end of the surgery and the strongest possible immune system to fight the underlying illness.
- Yoga and meditation have been proven to boost the immune system by around 30 per cent.
- One study showed that people with a God or people with religious beliefs, like for like, live on average seven years longer than the norm. Another showed that people who attend church regularly live on average seven years longer than those who don't. At Dukes in Carolina, doctors have recently noticed that those sufferers who believe in a God do indeed survive longer, and they are about to conduct specific research into this finding.

All of the above indicate that there are healing factors well beyond those normally considered by Western medicine. I am not saying use alternative medicine instead of radiotherapy. By and large radiotherapy does knock back cancers. The question is, can we use broader based therapies beyond those of Western science to help improve rates for cancer cure or to prevent cancer in the first place? And the answer is, undoubtedly, YES!

Macmillan Cancer Relief has recently launched *The Directory of Cancer Self Help and Support*, it lists over 700 local cancer support groups and organisations throughout the UK. It provides information on how to access self-help and support groups that offer assistance to people living with cancer, their partners, families and friends, and people bereaved through cancer. See appendix III for further details

Q29. What other factors can affect my general health and well-being?

In the West, orthodox medicine envisages the body as a machine where we are now able to remove a part such as a heart or kidney that is not functioning properly and replace it. The case for cloning that is argued in the media and by governments, is that scientists could end up with a perfect set of spare parts for each of us if and when something breaks down.

What if we were more than a complex set of machine parts? What if each of our mechanical parts was imbued with an over-riding system that was uniquely ours? What if this over-riding system was more powerful in terms of our health than the mechanical part?

Each of us has a body energy system unique to us.

There are three models of this. One from China that spread throughout the Far East, one that had its origin in India and a third developed relatively recently in the West.

The Western version is very similar to the Indian model. Around your body there are seven layers of energy fields that each have their own frequency, colour, density and fluidity and together form your aura. We know they exist!

A Russian, Kirlian, developed a method of photographing this aura 30 or so years ago. American scientists have done a lot of work on this in recent years measuring it, weighing it and studying, in particular, how two people might communicate between their auras. The frequency of the energy fields and the colours they emit change with the mood of the individual, for example, if they are angry or being untruthful, and with their health.

The seven layers each come from one of seven points on your body, each being a spinning vortex of energy called a chakra, down the centre line of your body.

The first layer is linked to your first chakra at the base of your spine, the second to your sacrum, the third to your solar plexus, the fourth to your heart, the fifth to your throat, the sixth to your forehead and the seventh to your crown. Each also links to an organ in the endocrine system eg the sixth to the pineal gland. The first three chakras are concerned with elements of your physical being like practicality or emotion, the fourth is connected to the heart and associated with love, whilst the outermost, highest three layers are linked to the spiritual plane.

You can have auric pictures taken of your fingertips which not only show aura lines radiating out from them, but the nerve endings connected (depending upon the finger and the position) to each of the body's organs. If there are toxins in the organ, the colour of the auric lines actually changes and can be used for diagnosis. I know, I've seen mine and the diagnosis was spot on!

When you lose someone you love dearly, poets would like us to believe you suffer a broken heart. But actually it is the chakra of emotion that suffers, giving you a painful sensation not in the heart region but in the solar plexus at the top of the stomach.

Our energy layers interact with those of other people just as the magnetic fields interacted when we saw experiments with magnets and iron filings at school. And we know that some people make us happy to be with them, while others simply drain our energy.

Our energy levels interact with our environment. A bird singing may calm us, a warm bath will relax us (it temporarily reduces our auric field), the sound of a glass window pane breaking at four in the morning may frighten us, a storm may stress us. American scientists have studied the basis of these energy systems and proven that you have channels, which take the energy fields inside the body to the internal organs. The blocking of channels can lead to illness, and acupuncture works by unblocking these channels.

Illness is believed to start with your energy flow being weakened or disrupted. In other words your energy system becomes unbalanced and gets ill first.

Dr Richard Gerber in his book *Vibrational Medicine* said, *'From an energetic standpoint, the human body when weakened oscillates at a different and less harmonious frequency than when healthy. If the same individual is supplied with a dose of the needed energetic frequency it allows the cellular bioenergetic systems to resonate in the proper vibrational mode, thereby throwing off the illness'.*

Since your chakras link to:

- The practicalities of your life
- Your emotions
- Love (and your relationship with others)
- Your spiritual relationship with the universe.

All these things can, and do, make you ill. There are some people who are naturally full of energy. They seem to radiate it, whilst others are depressed and lifeless.

And so we have a picture building up, that your energy system is linked to your brain and your emotions, to your endocrine system and your hormones, to your nervous system and to your internal organs. And to the universe around each of us.

Clearly, then, all of us who want to prevent or cure a cancer need to be aware of our own body energy and to do everything in our power to keep it flowing strongly and smoothly, ensuring that it is in balance and cleansed. All of us should on a regular basis see expert cranial osteopaths, acupuncturists, masseurs, reflexologists, reiki masters, homeopaths, aromatherapists; take your pick

Everybody should think of taking up yoga, t'ai chi or some other exercise that aims to regulate and improve the flow of energy in their bodies as a regular weekly habit. But be careful, you also just might enjoy it!

144

Q30. How important is my mental attitude?

Crucial.
Why is it that two patients with same affliction react so differently? One will take himself off to bed, while the other runs, plays sport, goes out and laughs it off.

Everybody stamps their condition with their own unique personality.

Death rates from cancer are higher among people in psychological distress and lower in people with a stronger sense of self-worth and self-purpose. Fact. Yet mechanically these people are the same. No wonder a doctor's work is so difficult.

Fear-motivated behaviour, guilt, depression, people who feel imperfect, inadequate, people who dwell in the past, who strive to be something they are not, people who judge others and themselves all the time, these people get ill.

In fact, people used to treating cancer patients describe a typical cancer sufferer as someone who 'tends to be a nice person, who wants to please and be liked. These people do not hold themselves in very high esteem and feel the cancer is somehow what they deserve'. The truth about these people is that with emotional scars and a feeling of always atoning for their sins or inadequacies, they don't nurture themselves enough, they don't respect themselves enough and they don't value themselves enough.

Cancer patients don't just need to change their physical lifestyle and diet, they need to change their mental attitude too.

Relax, be content with yourself, live in neither the past nor the future but here and now, don't apologise or feel guilty, be happy, have fun, love life, love yourself, think nice things, don't be habitually critical. Most importantly realise that you have strengths and skills, that you are a 'loved' person who deserves the best in life and has the ability deep inside you to be special.

'Our deepest fear is not that we are inadequate. Our deepest fear is that we are powerful beyond measure. It is our light, not our darkness, that most frightens us. We ask ourselves: "Who am

I to be brilliant, gorgeous, talented, fabulous?" Actually, who are you not to be? You are a child of God. Your playing small doesn't serve the world'. This was written by a man with every reason to be depressed and inadequate after years of imprisonment often fearing for his life and that he might never be free; Nelson Mandela.

In his book *The Road Less Travelled*, Scott Peck tells us to equate, 'Time with value with love'. If you love a baby you value it and you want to spend time with it. So too with yourself. Everyone must find time to love themselves and to show themselves that they value their life and being in good health. Time to shop properly for fresh produce or to cook nutritious foods, time to have a Thai massage, time to take exercise, time to be calm. Henry Kissinger once said, *'Next week there can't be any crisis; my schedule is already full.'* And that's the world we live in.

Stress, crises, unhappiness, fear of inadequacy, fear of failure are just some of the negative forces at work in our minds. Unfortunately the very people who have emotional problems are most prone to smoke and drink and not to look after themselves. This is less because of the pressure of work and practicalities, and more because of their emotional needs. If you can work on your emotional needs and fears, and strengthen your sense of purpose you will respect yourself more. Surely smoking heavily or pouring excess alcohol down your throat is a sign that you have little respect for yourself or your body.

Time magazine (20 January 2003) carried a 40 page special entitled 'How your mind can beat your body'. This collected the latest information from a huge number of sources.

It showed how, by using Positron-Emission Tomography or Functional Magnetic Resonance, pictures of the brain could be taken linking brain activity with diseases in different parts of the body. When you have a cancer in a certain part of your body, a shadow is observed on the part of the brain corresponding to that part of the body.

The brain is just one of many body organs and exhibits the same biochemistry as all the other organs. When the brain is depressed the biochemical activity of the cells in the brain exhibits certain characteristics. These are then communicated to the heart, lungs or breast and those cells will mirror the same biochemistry. Brain chemicals such as serotinin, for example, circulate throughout the body.

It is thus no surprise that people who are depressed have higher rates of heart disease and cancer. In November 2002 top experts in America met in Washington to discuss the evidence linking depression with disease. Depression is known to alter the structure of the blood making blood cells less likely to clump together. They carry less oxygen and this helps oxygen-hating cancer thrive, and they indirectly increase inflammation around the arteries.

Twenty per cent of diabetic women have depression, and depression makes the body less responsive to insulin. Insulin plays a role in cancer too. Depression affects cortisol levels and like insulin this stimulates localised bad eicosanoid production.

Stress results in the release of a flood of hormones in the body which affect nervous responses, organs and cellular biochemistry. Even low level stress is linked with low levels of circulating glucocorticoids, which in turn lead to a greatly weakened immune system.

Naturopathy and PNEI

Naturopathy is an ancient system of healing, which encourages building immunity naturally by viewing the individual as an integral part of nature's big picture.

Conventional medicine has recently overlapped with naturopathy through the study of Psycho-Neuro-Endocrino-Immunology or PNEI

Put simply: our feelings, emotions and thoughts are fundamentally connected to the working of our bodies.

PNEI is founded on two important principles:

- That in a hostile and toxic environment two people can differ completely in their susceptibility to illness. This is due, in naturopathic terms, to a personal and individual immunity; an inner profile.
- That there is a clear link between different emotions and both the nervous and endocrine system. Substances are then secreted, which actually affect receptor points on the cellular membrane

(probably through the eicosanoid system). So biochemically a stressful situation in your workplace 'stresses' your cells. A depressing meeting affects your mood and depresses your cells. A person who feels worthless has 'worthless' cells.

Both a healthy outer energy system and a strong inner profile provide immunity. But equally, a weakened energy system, or stressful emotional situations weaken your immunity. Not surprisingly people in continuous depressed states have been shown to have immune systems 30 per cent weaker than the norm.

Your mind is linked to your body energy. It is linked to your hormones and your nervous system and, through receptors, to your cells, and thus your cellular biochemistry.

So what can any of us do?

Firstly, as I have said, take time for yourself. Be idle, be calm, relax, meditate, take a massage, learn yoga. It is not a sin to do nothing. As Robert Louis Stevenson said, *'To be idle requires a strong sense of personal identity.'*

Secondly, as any good life coach will tell you, achieving a better life is not always about setting goals and striving. There is more often the need to remove from your life those things or people that limit you, or hold you back, or cause you most stress and pain.

There are too many people in this world who try to make you feel guilty or smaller or subservient. This is because they cannot generate their own vital energy and need to draw it from others. If you have a colleague, friend or even partner who does this, you must recognise that ultimately it may make you ill, and act accordingly. Start by analysing yourself. What causes you hurt, distress or pain; which people criticise you unfairly or make you feel guilty? Cut these things and these people out of your life for your health's sake. This is the first step to rebuilding your self-esteem.

It is a well studied fact that all animals and people are either providers or takers of energy. By and large children and animals are takers of energy. Large dogs and horses are providers of energy, adult humans can be either providers or takers depending upon their emotional background and stability.

Surround yourself with a real support group. Optimists, positive thinkers, happy people, people with their own energy, vitality and ideas. Avoid the pessimists, the critics and the moaners.

Where you cannot remove extreme emotional stress after, say, the loss of a close family member, you have to put it in the context of your own life and try to be positive about it. Counselling or visualisation, especially if you are seriously ill, may well be a good idea.

To best avoid illness you must have a strong sense of purpose about your own life. This is often quite weak in cancer sufferers, many of whom like spend more time trying to please those around them, or doing things to impress and gain plaudits rather than seeking things that make them happy themselves. Eventually, of course, these people end up not being true to themselves.

To be at your healthiest you need to have:

• An honest understanding of your own strengths and weaknesses
• An honest understanding of your own identity, your likes and dislikes
• A sense of purpose which genuinely reflects the above and is yours and not modified by other people's desires for you.

Be at peace with yourself. You have wonderful strengths so start to recognise them and appreciate yourself. Be positive in all your beliefs. Develop the 'I can do it' mentality. As Henry Ford said, *'Whether you think you can or you think you cannot, you are usually right!'* Be in no doubt that you are physically the summation of how you feel about yourself.

Naturopathy is at the basis of most alternative health treatments. It holds a number of fundamental tenets:

• Health is psycho-physiological. The distinction between mind and body is artificial. The more physical the symptom, the more psychologically accented needs to be the treatment.
• Health is nutrition. You are what you eat. If your crops failed to grow you would look to their nutrients, from soil to rainfall. So too with your body.
• Health is movement. Movement and posture increase natural

energy flow, improve circulation and the health of the internal organs, dissipate nervous energy and toxins.

- Health is concerned with the quality of life not merely the duration.

Naturopathy holds a simple belief that the body has the power to heal itself. When your body is in pain your tears show evidence of the endocrine system starting the healing process. Modern medicine overrides this, giving counter-action medicines such as antibiotics, anti-inflammatories and antidepressants. This approach, called allopathy, is directed against the signs or symptoms of the disease. It is not intended to find the root cause, the underlying problem, merely to cover up the symptoms in the hope that that is enough.

But if you want to prevent cancer it is imperative you work on your underlying health.

Cancer is the symptom of another illness; one which may have started even now to overtake your greater body and one you must address if you really want to beat it.

All of this can be summarised as follows:

A healthy body starts with a happy attitude, a sense of purpose, and a total feeling of self worth and value. This feeling in itself directly stimulates the nervous and endocrine systems, making your immune system and your cellular biochemistry stronger. This will in turn make you happier and lead you to value yourself more, for example, in your approach to your life, friends and work or in taking exercise, in taking time for yourself, in choosing what you should or shouldn't eat. This in turn further stimulates the immune system and builds your body energy. This is the way to beat cancer, and indeed all illness.

Q31. How can I revitalise my energy?

In Eastern philosophies energy systems are seen as a reflection of the universe, and are influenced by diet, climate and environment plus mental and spiritual attitudes.

Chi (in China), ki (in Japan) and prana (in India) are words for energy. Hence rei ki is Universal Energy.

Chi (also known as qi) is the Chinese term for 'vital energy' and enters the body through the air we breathe and the food we eat. Poor, unclean air and poor breathing habits such as shallow breathing both result in imbalance and thus illness.

Chi flows through the body along a network of channels, the meridians. There are 12 major ones, most linking to an organ in the body. Each meridian has a channel on either side of the body. Yang energy comes from the sun and flows down the body, yin comes from the earth and flows up the body.

If a person is unhealthy the energy flow is uneven, disturbed or even blocked. We all know that the wrist has a pulse for the blood system. At almost the same point each wrist has three pulse points for energy, each corresponding to certain organs, so that six organs in total are represented.

Most of the effective methods of revitalising energy come from Eastern philosophies. Here are some examples:

Qigong

Over 60 million Chinese use qigong which develops a body's energy in four ways – breathing, movement, body stance or posture and meditation. Exercise, breathing and posture develop the body's energy and flow whilst specific exercises can be used to unblock meridians

T'ai chi

Millions of people practise t'ai chi each morning. Graceful, physical movements and breathing combine with balance to improve the circulation, open up the lymph systems and the flow of vital energy, in turn stimulating the immune system. T'ai chi exercises stem from qigong, with the emphasis being on the mind, relaxation and internal energy rather than external energy development. As well as being a beneficial set of exercises, tai chi also has martial applications and can be an effective form of self-defence.

Reiki

Reiki is a form of 'hands on' healing where a reiki master imparts universal energy into your chakras; he or she is merely a conduit for that energy. In traditional Japanese medicine ki 'lives' about one inch below the navel and it is here all the energy for the body's support systems finds its roots. The reiki master's hands will often appear very hot (you lie down fully clothed) and you may 'see' flashes of coloured lights even though your eyes are shut. Expert reiki masters are definitely worth a visit and they can recharge you and get your energy flowing again. Reiki masters believe that everyone has the power naturally within them to transmit universal energy and affect another's body energy.

Cranial osteopathy

Cranial osteopaths use the chakras and the line of the backbone to balance energy along the body, often moving energy from one area to another. They will look for blockage which can often be linked to skeletal problems and rebuild the flow and the energy levels where you need it by manipulation of both the skeletal system and energy states. It is well worth seeing a top class cranial osteopath every three months or so for a body energy and skeletal service.

Yoga

Yoga has extraordinary benefits if it is done properly. A great many people know of its ability to increase flexibility but this is just one of its benefits. Yoga aims to affect two important aspects of your body:

• The link between your breathing, your mind and the control of energy into your body
• The opening of the energy channels and chakras to allow maximum flow between them and the internal organs.

Yoga's excellent at releasing and cleansing toxins from the body.

Ashtanga yoga is quite an athletic form of yoga perhaps better for younger readers as it involves higher than usual heart rates with exercises that are particularly strong on lymphatic drainage and stretching the body to stimulate the lymphatic system. However all yoga exercises can have a significant effect on unblocking chakras and on the immune system in general.

Pranayama is essentially breathing exercise. There are 72,000 channels or nadis in the body along which energy needs to flow freely for good health. Positions are adopted that link with breath control and these positions help open up channels.

Pranic breathing helps to correct poor breathing habits and encourages the flow of prana purifying the body. We Westerners breathe improperly only using about one third of our lung capacity so that our lungs always carry around stale air and toxins in their lower reaches. Correct breathing comes from correct posture, and using the abdominal muscles to force the diaphragm up and down. It does not come from chest expansion. Masters of this form of yoga 'breathe' in energy through their crown chakra. The process starts re-energising the root chakra and moves up the body through the seven chakras. When all seven chakras are so energised the body reaches its ultimate state of meditation.

Meditation

For some readers, it may seem hard to believe that meditation can actually re-energise you.

Remember that the energy systems, the mind, your breathing, your endocrine system, your nervous system, your blood and your lymph are all linked. Yogis believe that breathing exercises strengthen the body, clear the mind, maintain inner balance and thus help to prevent illness.

State of mind and breathing patterns are known to be linked, for instance, an agitated mind can result in rapid, shallow breathing.

By focusing attention on our breathing it can be gradually slowed and made deeper. This has a calming effect on the whole body and brain. Research has shown that the vibrational frequency of the brain waves changes, with different and slower frequency waves appearing during meditation. This in turn affects the endocrine system. Meditation has a profound effect on reducing cortisol levels which in turn lowers the levels of bad eicosanoids and promotes the levels of good ones. Meditation may involve constant chanting of a word or a noise. To stop the mind wandering you may add a constant theme or thought, for example love, as a focus. This in turn causes the release of favourable hormones inside the body.

Research tests on people who participate in yoga and meditation show higher outer energy states, and immune systems up to 30 per cent stronger than normal.

There is some evidence from Australia that meditation alone can lead to some remarkable cases of cancer healing. It certainly reduces blood pressure and resting heart rate.

Massage

Shiatsu, a Japanese form of massage, involves a professional practitioner examining the flow of energy along the meridians and using deep finger pressure at 'acupoints' to stimulate and regulate it. This benefits the lymph and nervous systems. There is a lot of overlap here with acupuncture, and shiatsu is an approved medical therapy in Japan.

Thai massage traces the lymph system in the body and stimulates its free flow. Like shiatsu, Thai massage involves deep, penetrating finger pressure. Lymph drainage is a term you have probably heard. After massage you must drink plenty of water as toxins will be 'turned out' of the lymph system.

Reflexology

The hands and feet are sites of nerve endings connected to all parts of the body. Sadly, a lot of reflexology resembles a nice foot rub. Done properly it can be diagnostic and re-energising as it helps to remove crystals and blockages, and stimulates the nervous system. These crystals are in fact toxins, which due to gravity, fall to the feet rather than being expelled from the body. If crystals are located, they can be massaged, broken up and then more easily expelled from the body, re-energising the corresponding organ and its blood supply. This can be a little painful depending upon the amount of crystals found.

Acupuncture

Acupuncturists gauge the strength of energy flow through the meridians by checking the six pulses in your wrists, each of which corresponds to an organ in your body. Along each meridian lie acupoints and by inserting a fine needle in some of them, blockages can be removed and a strong energy flow re-established to where it is needed. And, yes, you do feel the needles!

During both acupuncture and cranial osteopathy, you may feel tingling sensations as if water is flowing inside you. If you were particularly out of balance before, you may feel light-headed when you stand, something that can happen with reiki as well.

Acupuncture is now recognised as an important treatment by the medical services in both the USA and the UK.

Exercise

This form of re-energising the body is obviously not linked to Eastern philosophy but research evidence is clear. Exercise helps beat cancer.

Exercise strengthens the heart, the blood system, the lymph system and the skeletal structure. It clears toxins from the lungs, the cells and the blood. It releases 'happy' endorphin hormones, which neutralise negative hormones like adrenaline and it has a hundred other benefits. You are an animal – you are supposed to exercise. No other animal in its natural habit sits on chairs or works at computers.

Anybody who has been to China knows they cycle everywhere, so maybe it is not just the high selenium in their diet and dislike of dairy that keeps them cancer free!

However, walking to the station, a round of golf, making the beds or whatever the tabloids say this week does not officially qualify as exercise, that is, according to the UK Government. Their recommendation is as follows: for 20 minutes, three times per week, you need your heart rate to be between 55 per cent and 85 per cent of its theoretical maximum, which is 220 minus your age.

So, for example, a 50 year old has a maximum of 170 and 85 per cent is about 145. Non-stop, 20 minutes. Before that you warm up and afterwards you cool down.

As both a biochemist and a qualified personal trainer, I feel this is inadequate. Your fitness requirement has a need to stimulate the heart, the peripheral blood system and particularly the more passive lymph system. But this needs to be done every day not three times per week for 20 minutes.

One school of thought says that, through exercise, you should burn about 3,300 calories per week, which represents one and a half days normal calorie intake for a man. This equates to approximately 470 calories per day, which is about an hour on a bicycle each day. This should be even, calm exercise with the body constantly re-hydrated so that toxins can be taken away. You should eat protein within two hours after exercising and, during the whole process, you should be in control and able to talk without pause. This is a long way from the 'burn' of aerobics or an hour on a squash court. In fact extreme exercise, where you are out of breath and dehydrated, releases lots of toxins which the body must then remove from the cells, so beware. It makes far more of a case for t'ai chi than for a Jane Fonda style aerobics blast.

Finally, especially as you age, you need to do some resistance training. Lifting weights keeps up bone density avoiding brittle bones, so there is no need for women to take oestrogen in HRT. Go the gym instead. Lifting weights until they tire you also helps release a little growth hormone about 20 minutes after you finish This will mop up some free radicals and improve muscle tone and posture allowing energy to flow around the body better.

Two words of warning. Firstly, if you are over the age of 40, do not suddenly take up exercise or rekindle your sporting ambitions of 20 years ago. Work yourself back gradually ideally using a one on one expert or within a professional class. Secondly, drink plenty of water and keep yourself hydrated. If you feel dizzy, stop.

It is interesting to note that researchers at Bristol University have found that physical activity could significantly reduce the risk of bowel cancer by between 40 and 50 per cent and can help in the prevention of breast, prostate, lung and endometrial cancer. They are now studying the positive benefits of exercise for those people undergoing cancer treatment.

Indeed, Cancer Research UK sponsored a study by Bristol of all the worldwide research on exercise and cancer and from 54 studies the conclusion was drawn that exercise can prevent a cancer, and exercise can help recovery.

In summary

I hope this very limited summary of ways of cleansing your body and re-energising it, will have stressed the need to regard the body as much more than the sum of the physical parts. And to help you realise that t'ai chi or reflexology are not cranky mystical hocus pocus but can make a significant contribution to your body energy, endocrine and immune systems and therefore to cancer prevention and cancer cure.

There are many more holistic treatments, for example crystal healing, and both the Bristol Centre or the Hale Clinic in the UK will be able to impart more information. Suitable books and contact numbers are in the appendices.

Q32. Can homeopathy help?

Strictly speaking, homeopathy does not make any claims where cancer is concerned.

One branch of homeopathy, homotoxicology, looks at disease in six phases of which the first three phases have a favourable prognosis while phases four to six are less favourable but certainly not incurable. Cancer is, however, phase six.

In the average homeopathic practice most patients will come during or after orthodox treatment. Homeopathy can help a cancer sufferer in several ways:

- Firstly, homeopathy can help change someone's mental framework, for example, making them feel less suppressed by their surroundings and more positive with more self esteem.
- Secondly, homeopathy can help eradicate any parasites involved and, in certain cases, boost the body's immune system to fight off any virus that may be present. If you have a parasite or a virus, it can be identified by using EAV (electro-acupuncture according to Voll). Nosodes, best described as natural remedies that help stimulate the body's specific defences to that particular toxin, can be prescribed and the parasite or virus successfully eliminated.
- Thirdly, homeopathy can help detoxify and cleanse, antidote certain toxins, support specific organs and lift the overall body energy, or 'life force'.

In certain cases homeopathy can set up a reaction in the body to reinforce its ability to fight a specific cancer. There are specific nosodes to take for a number of cancers. For example, there is a nosode for brain tumours, and a homeopath I know treated herself and successfully beat breast cancer without radiation or chemotherapy.

It can be an aid during surgery, for example, to decrease bruising.

Finally, it can play a huge supporting role when patients are undergoing radio or chemotherapy. By supporting at the physical level, it helps patients withstand the depleting side effects and increases the effectiveness of both treatments.

Apart from its role with parasites and infections, homeopathy is not particularly relevant for prevention, which is felt to be more a role for diet and lifestyle changes. But if you have a cancer, homeopathy can form a part of a holistic approach to treatment.

As with modern medicine you must find a homeopath who has regular and specific experience of your type of cancer. This can be done through the Society of Homeopaths. Be very choosy. You'd only want the best brain surgeon, don't accept less in your homeopath.

Q33. How can I live a longer life?

Celebrate life; celebrate living

People who are in love have stronger immune systems. People who laugh a lot have stronger immune systems. Women who have regular orgasms have stronger immune systems. Smiling, happiness and joy all release certain beneficial hormones inside the body and these affect your nervous system, your lymph, your immune system and your whole well-being.

Positive thoughts, happiness and love radiate. The third and fourth chakras actually extend outwards, and two people who are deeply in love can have joined chakras. Even first encounters across a cocktail party have been observed with extensions of the third, the solar plexus, the emotional chakra!

Shouldn't you try to radiate more good vibrations? Try it and see what comes back your way. Maybe we can only see this through our sixth sense rather than through our eyes, but it still affects all our relationships. 'You only get back what you put in', or 'what goes round comes round,' would be two more common expressions.

J D Salinger once said, *'I am a kind of paranoic in reverse. I suspect people of plotting to make me happy!'* People will extend their energy systems towards you, if you do towards them.

The mention of spirituality in a book often finds people skipping a few pages: 'What has it got to do with me?' In a Western world that has turned its back on churches, the soul and the mere mention of God, it is all a bit too 'heavy' and often makes us feel a little uncomfortable because we have, in truth, dismissed most of it without too much thought.

But you exist as a mass of spinning electrons and you do have three layers of auric energy that connect you to the universe. A universe that itself is made of energy and is interconnected, so your well-being is inexorably linked with that universe and indeed the energy systems of the trees, plants and other animals around you.

Naturopaths do not view death as the end of life but merely as a part of our everyday lives since it occurs daily in our cellular system. Inevitably, though, all our cells die pretty much simultaneously.

However, given a simple Newtonian principle we all learned at school that 'energy can neither be created nor destroyed', what happens to our energy when we die? Officially, death may be when our heart stops, or our brain ceases to function, but hasn't it got something to do with our energy leaving our mechanical being?

One of the reasons for growing your own vegetables and eating them raw is that apart from getting all the vitamins and minerals untainted and undiminished you actually ingest their 'fresh' energy systems. A pea picked fresh is steamed in two minutes because it contains natural sugars. Kept for three days, molecular change has occurred together with a loss of energy and the sugar has turned to starch, requiring 20 minutes of steaming to cook it. **Fresh is not just about vitamins and minerals, it is about structure and energetic atoms.**

Understanding that the universe will nurture you by providing fresh energy, or stimulate or depress you through the interface with other people's energy systems is an aspect of spirituality. In Dukes, in Carolina, the doctors have noticed that two groups of people with cancer live longer. Those who fight, and those who have a God.

There is a strong argument that the higher success rates in cancer treatment in America over Britain are in part due to a determination not to accept the status quo, to demand second opinions and alternative diagnoses. This fighting spirit is in contrast to an often resigned apathy amongst British patients who leave themselves in the hands of their doctor. Having a fighting spirit is not being a 'pain in the arse', it's about being true to yourself.

Having a God is about being at peace with yourself. Several different studies show that people with a God and people who regularly attend church have longer lives, probably because their beliefs allow them the thought that God is supporting them, which results in them having a happier, more positive mental outlook.

In neither case do you have the stress of being something you

161

are not. Being untrue to yourself does not just make you ill, it is something other people can perceive from your aura, and so it negatively influences their relationship with you.

Inside your energy system you have a core; the Chinese talk about meridians, the ancient Egyptians about a merkaba, Christians about your soul, and the Japanese about the centre of ki. Even if you are not religious the appropriateness of the biblical statement, '*What good will it be for a man if he gains the whole world, yet forfeits his soul?*' (Mathew 16:26) seems exceptionally relevant in this modern world.

We live in a world where all manner of modern day sins pull us in the wrong direction, whether they are alcohol, drugs, gorgeous meals, late night parties or over indulgence. Perhaps we have to ensure that we nourish our souls as much as our physical bodies by appreciating the natural world around us a little more. And we should take the time to do this.

Spirituality is about strengthening our total being (and yes ultimately our immune system), cuddling our children, trying to understand the needs of others, performing acts of kindness, being happy, being trustworthy, truthful, sincere, true to ourselves and so on. Kirlian photography has shown that yogis have much larger auras, which are the product of their humble yet generous spiritual lifestyles, not solely of the physical benefits of yoga.

Spirituality is not confined to a link with a greater energy, God and the universe, death and the after life. It is about the life in your days rather than the days in your life. It's about the life inside you. And the life inside you that can protect and cure you from cancer.

SECTION IV

What do I do if I get cancer?

Important

This section includes tips and advice gleaned from a number of expert sources.

However before embarking on any course of action, or refraining from any action, readers are advised to consult with their own expert practitioner.

The following section must only be viewed as suggestion and nothing more. Neither the author or publisher can be held responsible for any actions taken or avoided as a result of information contained here.

Q34. If I get cancer, what should I do?

People say that when they first hear that six-letter word their head spins and so many thoughts rush through their mind that they miss most of what is then said. 'Will I die?' is the most common thought. The answer to this is very likely 'no', but it is about odds. Right from the first moment you must start trying to improve yours.

Doctors talk about five year survival rates; 150 per 1,000 with lung cancer, 850 per 1,000 with breast cancer. But, of course, that is an average. If you are young, don't smoke and do everything in your power to increase your odds your chances will be much better.

Remember three out of four people on average survive. Don't be average, be better.

- The NHS cancer referal guidelines (agreed in 2000) state that any patient who has a sign or symptom that could be caused by cancer, has to be referred to a specialist within two weeks.
- At the first consultation have someone with you (your 'buddy') and prepare a list of questions to take with you. Take notes, have a tape recorder (ask first but there should be no problem) and let your buddy ask questions too. Agree with the consultant a convenient time for a further question and answer session because you will get home and find that new questions spring to mind, partly because oncologists 'cushion' the answers to questions for fear of upset, and often seem evasive.
- Ask for your medical notes. Since November 1991 you have a right to see all notes and correspondence relating to your case.
- Find out exactly what the plan is for your recovery, what treatment is to be recommended. Ask about likely problems, how success will be assessed (eg complete recovery in six months, going back to work), and what chances there are of the cancer recurring.
- Look into other sources of information and help.

- contact the Bristol Cancer Help Centre for their dietary advice for your particular cancer, together with advice on other alternative treatments you can start immediately

- phone the Macmillan Cancer Relief's helpline or the Cancer BACUP and ask specifically for the phone number of the help group relating to your particular cancer
- find a friend who is good on the internet and ask them to help you access your cancer type, looking for any drugs recommended so that you and your buddy can keep informed with absolutely up to the minute information
- go to www.cancerhelp.org.uk for all the latest news and help in simple, plain English
- only go to experts and demand the best in whatever field you use
- ask for a second opinion
- keep focused on what you are going to do when you recover. Think about your new life, new diet and new sense of purpose
- read this book carefully and keep it to refer to

• Other questions you might want answered are:

- what help and care will Social Services provide?
- am I eligible for any government financial help? Or from any cancer or other charitable organisations?
- how will this affect my private healthcare or my life insurance?
- what difference would it make if I went privately and what would it cost?
- where is the best place and where are the best doctors for my type of cancer?
- is this treatment likely to make me infertile? If so can I do anything about it or about preserving my sperm or eggs?

Doctors have a system for defining how bad the cancer is. You should ask, 'is it a primary and do I have secondaries?'. Cancers are defined in terms of 'grade' and 'stage', each on a 0–4 scale. After a biopsy (or sample) of the tumour is taken, you should be told what 'grade' the cancer is. Low-grade tumours are slower growing and considered less dangerous, but high-grade tumours are deemed aggressive.

The spread of the cancer from its origin is deemed the stage. With a breast cancer for example the spread may be a long way, maybe to the lymph nodes. The maximum grade is 4, meaning widely disseminated. Cancer may spread via the blood or lymph systems.

In the case of many tumours, a lung or whole body X-ray or scan will be taken to see whether the tumour is a primary, or a secondary to a primary in another location.

Finally, blood tests will in several cases show evidence of tumours (eg prostate cancer). All this should all be confirmed in a written histology report and you are entitled to a copy. Get hold of this, read it, discuss it with your buddy and your specialist and write an action plan (see next question).

You cannot know too much. Information is power. Remember, in the USA the survival rates are higher than in the UK and one of the major reasons for this, since the treatments themselves are often comparable, is the sheer determination and fighting spirit of the American sufferer. They argue more, demand second opinions, new medicines and drug trials, whatever it takes. The fighting spirit carries them forward and, the fact is, keeps them alive longer. Apparently British sufferers are far too accepting of their fate, 'I have cancer, it's a life-threatening situation but my doctor will do his best for me'.

Do not be like this.

Be determined. Be a fighter and be positive.

Q35. How do I improve my chances of being cured?

Three quarters of all cancer sufferers in Britain are cured. The definition of a cure used by the medical profession is that the patient did not die from their cancer within five years of being diagnosed.

So, three out of four people with cancer will survive. As I said at the start, the moment you are diagnosed you should immediately start to think:

'How can I improve my odds?'
'How can I move the 75 per cent figure to 100 per cent for me personally?'
Start taking action immediately putting in place the following 'action plan', referring to summary 3 in section V and reading the relevant sections of this book:

- Evaluate your diet, and go on to a strict diet as outlined

- Take a crash course of supplements

- Evaluate your lifestyle
- cut out carcinogens, like drinking, smoking and cosmetics
- take exercise; try yoga and meditation.

- Get support
- contact the cancer helplines
- talk to cranial osteopaths, homeopaths, acupuncturists, visualisers, healers
- have a virus, parasite and yeast check.

- Concentrate on you
- cut all the stresses from your life, be absolutely ruthless about this
- take time for yourself
- find a buddy who will stick with you throughout.

- Be determined
- be absolutely clear. This is a fight to the death. The death of

you or the death of the cancer, and the odds already say you should win. But be determined, be disciplined and really do exactly what is necessary to beat it without cutting corners or making compromises.

- Focus on the future
- when I have beaten this, how is my life going to change? Who do I want to be? What do I want to do? What would I like to have? What would I like to learn?
- give yourself clear and attainable reasons for living and focus on them. Don't just settle for more of the past. Think about your personal development.

Make no mistake, you were no victim unless there was a severe attack of asbestos from your roof, or a leak from the nuclear power station nearby! By and large you contracted cancer because of your own personal habits. Plan ahead, plan to change them to make yourself well, and start now planning the new life you want in five years' time.

The medical profession will now swing into action and it will all happen expertly and very, very quickly. Sometimes it seems, too quickly. Now is the time to plan. Three treatments are the likely options:

- Surgery
- Radiotherapy
- Chemotherapy.

I will deal with each in turn in the following pages.

It may only be days before your surgery. It may be four to 10 weeks before radio or chemotherapy, depending upon the region you are living in and whether you are NHS or private.

Use the time wisely for both short-term and long-term preparation.

Q36. What about a second opinion?

Firstly, let me concentrate on the first opinion. Biopsy plus CT or MRI scan and blood tests should give a clear picture of the problem.

- A computed axial tomography (CT or CAT) scan is a 3 D X-ray and takes 20–30 minutes.
- A Magnetic Resonance Imaging (MRI) scan uses a magnetic field instead of X-rays and takes about 30 minutes. Both CTs and MRIs produce a clear and accurate picture of the scene around the tumour and a dye might be injected to show the tumour up more clearly.
- X-rays of other areas of the body may then be taken to discover if there is only one tumour. Armed with all this information ask the doctor in front of you if they are going to manage your whole recovery process, which may involve surgery, neurology, radiotherapy and chemotherapy. If they are not, then who is?

In the field of cancer, where several treatment options are possible and clearly the patient is in a life threatening situation, it is considered the norm to ask for a second opinion and all the medical records should be made freely available to the patient to pass on to a second expert. It will definitely not be seen as a vote of no confidence, in fact a second opinion is a natural, concerned and intelligent thing to embark on. Your doctor will actually expect you to be interested enough in your own personal welfare to be taking a second opinion, and that second opinion, even if it reaches the same conclusion as the first one, should help you feel more confident about the complete process of treatment.

So how do you find a second opinion?

- You can ask your GP, but they have more than likely referred you to the person they consider to be the best in the first place. You could go to a private GP and ask what they think and for their views on other sources.
- You can search the internet. Many acclaimed international hospitals offer a simple 'send us the information' service.

- Try to get the second opinion from outside of the system that gave you the first. Doctors trained in the same hospital will usually give you the same answers.
- You can telephone a large teaching hospital which will help you establish the top specialists in your type of cancer.
- You can go for a second opinion to the alternative medicine field. If you do, go to someone with a lot of experience in your specific cancer.

Having taken a second opinion discuss it with your original doctor and again prepare an action plan with your buddy.

Q37. Can you tell me about surgery?

Approximately 60 per cent of cancer patients will have surgery. However, it can take several forms.

Some operations may involve **endoscopes** where an instrument is inserted through a hole made in the body. The endoscope allows the surgeon to 'see' inside the body and take a small amount of tissue for examination.

Some operations may involve a similarly small treatment. For example, the majority of bladder cancer only affects the bladder lining and can be removed using a **cytoscope** (a tube passed into the bladder). The bladder can continue to work normally and, even if the cancer returns, it may be possible to work on it again in this way.

Some operations, whilst requiring the surgeon to open up the body, may only be to take tissue for testing. For example, in cases of brain tumours the surgeon may open up the skull, take some tissue from the tumour, and then use titanium screws to hold the skull back in place. At a later date, if there is a need for a full operation, or a second operation, the plate can be lifted.

Surgery in these examples is **diagnostic**. The surgeon uses his skills and, with the aid of the pathology and histology reports, can make an accurate assessment of the problem.

It should be stressed that in the majority of these cases, the results will indicate that the problem is not malignant.

However, after taking samples for test, the tumour may be deemed malignant and the surgeon's role will be crucial in establishing the stage and/or grade of the cancer. Metastasis is the name given to the process by which malignant disease spreads to distant parts of the body, and to the secondary tumours resulting from this process. For example, the rogue cells can circulate in your blood stream to attack cells in your liver or brain, or it is possible that the body's natural defence system will have identified rogue cells and taken them via the lymph to the lymph nodes for examination.

If the tumour is confined to a single site and is whole, like a pea or a ball, it is said to be a **solid tumour**. This is ideal for surgery and the whole tumour may be removed effectively. For example breast, stomach, thyroid, testicular and skin cancers are often tackled in this way. If the primary has been detected early enough, the messages to other parts of the body may be minimal and surgery can be an effective one-stop cure.

If the tumour has started to spread, the surgeon may also remove some of the surrounding tissue. If it has moved to a lymph gland he may well remove that too.

These days, a surgeon would always prefer to confine his surgery to a localised removal eg breast lumps or bowel tumours, rather than having to perform radical extensive surgery. The former is clean and limited and considerably improves the quality of the patient's life.

If the cancer has spread, or there is a risk it may have done, surgery may well be followed by radiotherapy and/or chemotherapy. Further surgery is also a possibility but is only needed in a small number of cases.

There have been debates about whether the action of surgery itself causes the cancer to spread. There was a report in the *Lancet* in 1995 about this possibility with prostate cancer. Anyway the anaesthetic will flatten your immune system and make you more susceptible to the cancer spreading immediately after the surgery, so take positive action to boost your immune system with the ideas in this book.

Finally remember one important fact. The surgeon will do his level best to cut out all the cancer from your body that he safely can. But it is most likely that your diet, the products you use and your lifestyle brought on the cancer originally. You will ultimately only beat the cancer if you change the habits that gave it to you in the first place. For a short while your life may be in his hands. But in the longer term, it's in your own.

Q38. What should I ask the surgeon?

1. Please describe the operation in detail
2. What are the risks during the operation?
3. What are the risks after the operation?
4. Will surgery cure the problem or merely slow it down?
5. What does the surgeon consider to be success?
6. What are the short-term and long-term side effects?
7. What follow up would be needed after surgery?
8. What if my cancer comes back after surgery?
9. How often has the surgeon performed this particular operation before?

The most important thing is to get the best expertise. Common cancers may be treated by oncologists at the patient's local unit. Less common ones should be referred to specialist units and doctors who have a track record in the specific cancer.

It is possible to access the database at the Department of Health or your Local Strategic Health Authority to check out your surgeon. Don't be shy about this, it is your life after all!

Q39. What can I do to recover from surgery quickly?

- Likely scars can be lessened by taking the following supplements daily
  - 2 gms vitamin C (4 x 500 mgs Ester C, time release or at different times of the day)
  - 400 IU vitamin E (you can take up to 1,000 IU)
  - 25 mgs zinc
  - 1,000 mgs of cod liver oil.

- The above supplements may also help your immune system, but you could add the following daily to really boost it:
  - 6 mgs of beta-carotene twice per day
  - 200 mcgs of selenium
  - Drink 6–12 cups of Essiac per day
  - 10–20 mgs of lycopene
  - 30 mgs coenzyme Q10.

There are more suggestions in the answers in Section II.

- The following have an immune boosting effects and specific action on tumours:
  - 2 garlic tablets twice per day
  - 2 gms soya isoflavones per day
  - 2–3 gms astragalus per day.

- Drink 1.5–2.5 litres of good quality water per day to flush the anaesthetic through and take a three to five day detox·when you come out of hospital. Buy a simple herbal detox from a pharmacy and read the instructions or ask the pharmacist.

- Toxins can be removed from the alimentary canal by adding 2 tablespoons of linusit (organic linseeds) to your breakfast cereal and taking 1,500 mgs of psyllium seeds each day. If you increase your fibre intake you should increase your zinc intake to 50 mgs as fibre prevents zinc absorption, and you must drink lots of water with both.

- If the tumour was in the brain take 500–1,500 mgs of soya

lecithin per day as this contains choline and inositol, two B vitamins which cross the blood/brain barrier and nourish brain cells. Soya lecithin will help all your cell membranes, and your liver.

- Take a multivitamin and multimineral complex preferably in colloidal form and containing iron to help in blood regeneration. The B vitamins it contains will also help to overcome the stress of the operation and aid the healing process, for example, biotin will help the action of vitamin C and folic acid will help your DNA replicate correctly.

After the operation, massage the scar gently with vitamin E cream.

Manual lymphatic drainage (MLD)

- Lymphoedema is a chronic swelling due to a failure of lymph drainage. It can sometimes occur after cancer surgery where the adjacent lymph nodes have been removed or radiated. If the lymph nodes under the arm have been surgically removed following breast cancer, this can result in a swollen arm. After testicular or prostate cancer treatment, removal of the nodes in the groin can cause swollen legs or abdomen.
- Lymphoedema is not curable, and if left untreated can lead to many problems including, an increase in the size of the limb, or torso, and a hardening of the tissues (fibrosis), which can impede most of the lymph flow. The area becomes vulnerable to infection and can result in a painful inflammatory condition called cellulites.
- Manual lymphatic drainage (MLD) is an acknowledged therapy for helping to control and maintain lymphoedema, and is used together with skin care, exercises and breathing techniques. The therapist uses very gentle, precise hand movements to accelerate the flow of lymph through the lymphatic system. This results in a softening of the tissues, reduced swelling and a reduction in pain. When the normal drainage route has been destroyed by surgery or radiation it is possible to pump the lymphatic fluid towards functioning lymph vessels for them to take up the extra load, leading to a reduction of

the swelling. The gentle pumping action of MLD is used to great advantage to reduce the appearance of scars.

- When necessary, MLD is combined with compression bandaging and exercises designed to prevent the fluid returning to the area. After several treatments, dramatic improvements in swelling are often achieved. When the swelling has reduced, a maintenance programme of treatments is begun and the therapist can supply compression stockings or sleeves if needed. MLD is a deeply relaxing and soothing treatment.
- MLD therapists will give advice on treatment plans, skin care, exercises and self-massage where appropriate, and will liaise with the patient's doctor/consultant to ensure the best possible outcome. In the UK, there are several recognized training schools for MLD including Vodder, Asdonk, Le Duc, Foldi and Casely-Smith and it is vital that the therapist is properly trained.

Q40. Can you tell me about radiotherapy?

In an earlier answer the effect of free radicals damaging DNA was covered. If the configuration of the DNA is changed it is extremely likely that a nonsensical code sequence will be produced and the body's natural defence system will throw it out. Radiotherapy adopts the same principle, attempting to similarly change the DNA, albeit this time in a rogue cell, so that it becomes gobbledegook, is neutralised and similarly taken away by the body's natural defences.

Radiotherapy uses high speed ionising radiation similar to X-rays to hit the DNA in abnormal cells. To have an effect it must hit the DNA when it is dividing. Radiotherapy is very successful at screwing up this division, causing the copy to be full of errors. The radiation uses lasers fired from very large, very sophisticated machines and can be targeted very accurately.

The effectiveness of radiotherapy has to be balanced by the risks but, essentially, depending upon the grade, stage and type of cancer, radiotherapy works. It works during the programme of radiotherapy and for up to four to six weeks afterwards.

A little more detail

The higher the energy of the ionising rays, the deeper into the body the rays can go.

A package of energy is a 'photon' and this is divided into 'fractions'. Whilst X-rays were the first type used, these are now often replaced by gamma rays. Particle beam radiation using fast moving subatomic particles can also be used to treat localised cancers.

Internal radiotherapy involves placing small radioactive pellets or implants into the localised tumour to do the damage.

Techniques are being developed all the time in an attempt to kill more of the cancers' cells and less of the surrounding good guys. Radiosensitisers make the tumour more susceptible to damage from radiotherapy; radioprotectors protect the normal cells. Radio labelled antibodies are also being used as cancer seekers.

When treatment is considered, a patient will firstly go through a planning stage, lying under a simulator which takes X-rays of the area to be treated. In this way the medical team can target the tumour accurately and plan how to stay focused on that area, whilst moving the angle of attack to minimise damage to a healthy area adjacent to the tumour. Each session of radiotherapy is very short, just a few minutes, although radiotherapy may be required over a number of weeks. Radiotherapy is not painful.

The total dosage is very carefully calculated to do the most efficient and effective job so the patient must go to every planned session and avoid missing any. Apparently (and somewhat nonsensically) only about 20 per cent of patients go to all the treatments. One reason is the patient's depression, which is quite normal and can set in after a couple of weeks.

Sometimes one big dose is given rather than small does (stereotactic radiotherapy), depending upon the type of cancer and how far it has spread.

Radiotherapy is becoming more and more sophisticated, and is the medical profession's front line weapon in treating cancers effectively. It definitely does work but, because of the free radical action on the surrounding tissues, there is a small chance of contracting a second completely new cancer from the radiation itself. Ask about this.

Q41. What side-effects are there to radiotherapy?

These depend upon the exact type of cancer and the location.

- If the rogue cells are not dividing – and at any one time they will not all be doing so – they won't be affected.
- Other nearby healthy cells that are dividing can be damaged or killed. Often the healthy cells that are damaged belong to the blood supply system or membrane structure. The theory is that these normal cells will be regenerated in time, but this is not always the case. In the case of breast cancer, sometimes up to 15 per cent of lung tissue is permanently damaged in this way.
- The area may get a little 'burned', so bright sunshine on the skin should be avoided. The area attacked should be washed only in cold water and aloe vera gel used.
- Hair loss may well occur in the direct line of the beam but the hair will return.
- Radiation weakens the body overall. Both the blood and lymph cells are attacked by radiotherapy, reducing the numbers of both red and white blood cells. The liver also works overtime removing dead cells and toxins.
- Most patients get very tired and should plan to sleep or simply rest for a couple of hours per day. Fatigue can be a real problem and Italian doctors have identified the cause as low levels of carnitine circulating in the blood stream. They recommend taking energy drinks with supplements of carnitine. Apparently in research energy levels came back within one week for 90 per cent of patients. The tiredness will probably extend to lethargy and patients may also feel sick. Travelling long distances to the hospital may be tiring and the location of the treatment centre and its distance from where you stay the night need to be given some thought.
- Drinking peppermint tea may calm the stomach and help the nausea that affects some people.

The number of blood cells is called your blood count and this should be monitored carefully throughout radiotherapy. Radiotherapy must be stopped if the blood count falls too far.

- In extreme cases, radiotherapy can lead to sterility.
- Some people may suffer from mouth ulcers. If so, avoid all sugar and salt, calm your stomach with peppermint tea and avoid stress and acid foods.
- After about two weeks of treatment and again about two weeks after finishing treatment, the patient may suffer acute depression and it is at this point the buddy and family members, friends and partners need to rally round. Don't be embarrassed to ask someone to watch over you during this time. Going alone to radiotherapy in week three when you are tired and depressed can be a very lonely experience, so take someone with you. But you must keep up treatments and avoid missing any sessions.
- There is some evidence that radiotherapy, whilst it cures the first cancer, can cause long term problems in the surrounding healthy cells. Patients treated for cervical cancer can show major urinary problems 25 years later. Lung tissues are especially susceptible to radiation damage. In one research report, 19 of 31 breast cancer patients went on to get lung cancer, on average 17 years later.

Q42. What should I ask the doctor in charge?

1. What would the doctor consider to be a successful response at the end of the radiotherapy treatment?

   - no cancer tumour remaining?
   - tumour present but much smaller?
   - other?

2. How long will the treatment be? Will you be an outpatient or inpatient? Is this a one-off treatment, or might there be more?

3. What is the doctor's success rate, and how does that compare to the national average?

4. How often has the doctor personally treated your type of tumour?

5. What do they consider the next step after radiotherapy, and why?

6. What happens if there is no response? How often does that occur? What is the fallback plan?

7. What exactly do they think the side effects are likely to be?

8. What are the chances of each side effect?

9. What supplements would they recommend to improve

   - the success of the radiotherapy?
   - the reduction of side effects?
   - the speed of recovery?

Q43. How can I protect myself from the side-effects of radiotherapy?

We have already covered the fact that radiotherapy is going to attack all rapidly dividing cells in the line of fire. So it will attack the rapidly dividing cells adjacent to the cancer, flatten your blood count and lymph systems, and thus your immune system. It will fill the body, and especially the liver, with toxins and dead cells.

This means you have to have an action plan to try to keep yourself as strong as possible throughout. A major problem here is that some of the vitamins and supplements you might still wish to take to maintain your immune system will also inhibit the action of the radiotherapy by protecting the very cells it should be attacking.

Everything you can take is explained more fully in section II. So this section is intended to be little more than a checklist. From the start you should consider yoga and meditation, and using cranial osteopaths, acupuncturists and healers, to strengthen the immune system and aid your mind-energy-healing link.

It should be stressed up front, that three supplements in particular seem to have a proven record in making radiotherepy more effective. these are:

- Selenium
- Soya isoflavones
- Astragalus.

The suggested action plan divides into three stages and focuses on supplements as a way of kick-starting the health boosting plan. You may prefer to take less supplements and strengthen your diet in the ways I have previously outlined. A full diet is in section V.

(i) Pre-radiotherapy

As soon as you find out you have cancer you should:

- Go to a cranial osteopath and/or acupuncturist to balance and strengthen your body energy systems
- Start a yoga course and, if you feel up to it, maintain a light exercise programme. Learn to meditate.

- Take a multivitamin and mineral complex, ideally in a colloidal form, which includes some iron and B complex with at least 400 mcgs of folic acid
- Take

Beta-carotene	6 mgs twice per day
Vitamin C	500 mgs four times per day
Vitamin E	400 IU daily
Zinc	25 mgs daily
Selenium	200 mcgs daily
Coenzyme Q10	30 mgs daily
Lycopene	10–20 mgs daily

all of which will strengthen your immune system.

- Take 1,000 mgs of cod liver oil and 2 garlic tablets daily or eat lots of oily fish and raw garlic. Take 3,000 mgs astragalus and drink Essiac tea. Replace all drinks of tea, coffee and chocolate with green tea.
- Take an amino acid supplement containing glutamine. This stimulates the liver to produce glutathione, which is very strong in repairing damaged cells, and L-cysteine, which is particularly important in DNA repair. Alternatively, instead of taking the supplements, eat the foods in which they are naturally found. Glutathione is present in fruit and vegetables especially raw carrots, asparagus, avocado and cruciferous vegetables (eg Brussel sprouts, cabbage, broccoli). L-cysteine is found in kelp (seaweed), eggs and garlic.
- Switch away from all dairy products and use soya totally. Take 3 gms per day of soya lecithin, which has an excellent content of inositol and choline, as it is a fat emulsifier and will help the liver break down the excess fats lying there. Add to this 2 gms per day of soya isoflavones. This will help in all cases of hormone induced cancer.
- Detox. Buy a proprietary detox from a health store and use it for at least four days to help clean the liver.
- Drink 1.5–3 litres of pure water, which will also help clear away the toxins and clean the liver.
- Take 200 mgs per day of milk-thistle to strengthen your liver.

- Always avoid animal fats, saturated oils and dairy products as cancer cells thrive on fats.

(ii) During radiotherapy and for four to six weeks after

- Keep the momentum of the pre-radiotherapy stage going
- in terms of visits to the cranial osteopath/acupuncturist, regular yoga and meditation. But you will probably be too tired for regular light exercise
- take all the supplements except beta-carotene, vitamin C, lycopene, Cassie tea and coenzyme Q10, all of which might prevent the radiotherapy working properly. Take carnitine.
- ensure you do take the selenium, soya isoflavones and astragalus as all three have been proven to make radiotherapy work more effectively
- detox after three weeks, six weeks and nine weeks if you feel up to it
- continue drinking 1.5–3 litres of water and avoiding fats and oils.

This stage should continue for at least four to six weeks after the radiotherapy finishes as the action of the radiotherapy is still taking place although treatments have stopped. If you haven't felt up to it before, you should try to do a proper detox prior to starting Stage (iii).

(iii) Post-radiotherapy

- Keep all of the above going. Add back in the beta-carotene, vitamin C, lycopene and coenzyme Q10. Plus the Cassie tea.
- Take a supplement of organic iron for just one week at the start to raise your blood count.
- Take 1,500 mgs of echinacea and 1,000 mgs of cat's claw (Uno de Gato), the latter taken on an empty stomach, along with the 3,000 mgs of astragalus, all of which help to regenerate a healthy immune system quickly. See answer 19 for more details on herbal immune boosters.

Yes, you are taking a lot of pills, which you should spread out during the day. You can of course eat the natural alternative to some of the above and prepare wonderful fresh juices, but the supplement volumes above are 'insurance' amounts designed to give you the best possible chance of beating the cancer. A full diet plan is contained in section VI.

Q44. Can you tell me about chemotherapy?

Chemotherapy is the use of chemicals to poison rogue cells. Again it works on rapidly dividing cells, usually poisoning them through free radical toxic action.

The drugs used will vary according to the type of tumour and its state of advancement. Some chemicals work directly on the cell. Some work on the receptors at the cell surface and try to stop the rogue secondary messages getting through.

The risks are in the side effects. Chemotherapy is a very general treatment. Pills taken orally or drugs administered into veins poison the whole body. The liver and immune system do their best to remove the poisons, but both are weakened severely in the process. Other rapidly dividing cells, such as those in the nails, blood, stomach lining and hair, also suffer. Often sickness is a real problem, as it further debilitates the patient. During the chemotherapy the blood count declines and less oxygen is carried round the body. Often after a couple of weeks, and again around week six, the patient gets depressed. One reason is that the blood oxygen level and depression are directly linked. It can happen in reverse; depressed people have lower levels of oxygen carried in their blood streams.

Estimates suggest that, on average, 10 per cent of patients who undergo chemotherapy ultimately contract a completely new unrelated cancer at a later date, caused by the chemotherapy toxins damaging DNA in other cells. This estimate appears low according to recent research. Studies now show, for example, that one third of female childhood cancer survivors suffer a breast cancer by the time they are 40 years old. Indeed, amongst women in their late 20s and 30s, breast cancer is 16 times more common than the norm where chemotherapy was administered to them as children. Nearly one quarter of patients treated with anthracyclines go on to develop heart problems, with women being particularly affected.

In certain cancers the success rate of chemotherapy is as low as 1 per cent, and a survey of 128 US cancer doctors found that if they themselves contracted cancer over 80 per cent would not resort to chemotherapy as the, 'risks and side effects far outweighed the likely benefits'. What they would actually do if they had cancer is possibly another matter.

In a little more detail

Barely a week seems to go by without a new magic drug going through trials. No wonder in the USA alone the industry is a $7bn business.

There are a lot of drugs, all different and for different situations. Increasingly scientists are trying to localise the drug to the tumour. This is because when a pill is taken orally, or a drug intravenously, it spreads right round the body. The liver, for example, tries to expel it and so only a small percentage actually reaches the target; resulting in high wastage of the drug and random damage to the patient's body. This explains why the recipient can feel so ill, tired, depressed and why the liver and kidneys become so poisoned.

To illustrate current thinking and progress being made, here are some examples:

- Temozolomide is a new drug just given FDA approval to treat astrocytomas (Grade 3 brain tumours). It has been used on patients where the tumours have reappeared after radiotherapy and chemotherapy have failed. In tests amongst 54 patients, seven had tumours that shrunk and five had their tumours disappear. So a 9 per cent success rate and a 22 per cent effect. Possible side effects are headaches, nausea, fatigue and low blood counts.

- The FDA has approved a, 'wafer impregnated with a drug that is inserted next to the actual brain tumour'. This treatment, which fights Grade 4 glioblastoma multiforme and is called Gliadel, delivers the anti-cancer drug Carmustine directly to the tumour site in higher concentration. The six-month survival rate amongst 222 adults went up from 36 per cent with placebo to 56 per cent with Gliadel.

- There are trials being conducted in America using Toxin Therapy, for example, where a poisonous bacterium (in this case *Pseudomanas bacteriae*) is armed with an anti-cancer drug

(Interleukin 4) and only attacks and kills cancer cells but not the patient's healthy ones.

- Gleevec is a drug recently developed, which blocks a cellular receptor enzyme. When a rogue messenger hits a cell it has to be shunted through 58 receptors until it reaches the nucleus and can cause its havoc. Gleevec was developed to block that process. Although the drug was developed for use with brain tumours (it was originally called Glivac), it doesn't seem to work with them. However it was found to work with chronic myeloid leukaemia and the FDA has given its approval for the use of the drug with this disease.

By now you should be getting the picture. Vast effort, lots of different drugs, formats and applications. Low returns but increasing sophistication.

Do not rush in to chemotherapy without knowing all the facts. However, even some of these can be misleading. Doctors in the UK usually measure success as survival after five years. But although survival rates do vary by country so does the way survival is defined. In some countries a different figure is quoted, which is based on the number of people who did not die of the specific cancer within five years – this means that if a patient dies from a technically different disease, for example pneumonia, within the five years they can be included bizarrely in the survival column, even if the pneumonia was brought on by the cancer.

If your doctor recommends chemotherapy make sure you know everything about the drug he is suggesting. You will find new drugs covered on the internet complete with results of their trials. Or you can ask a professional complementary centre like the Bristol Cancer Centre or your specific cancer charity/foundation helpline and also get a second opinion. (The very latest cancer treatments can be obtained on the Medcast Web site – http://webmd-practice.medcast.com/smed/web).

Finally, a word of warning. Some complementary treatments, particularly diets and herbs, may affect the action of prescribed chemotherapy drugs. You should tell your specialist exactly what else you are doing for treatment and seek advice on possible reactions between the treatments.

189

Q45. What questions should I ask my doctor about chemotherapy?

1. How long has the doctor been prescribing this course of treatment, and how many people have undergone the treatment?
2. If they had your cancer, would they treat themselves with this drug?
3. How many cases have they treated with this drug, and what has the success rate been? (Define success!)
4. What are the alternatives?
5. What is the fall back if it doesn't work?
6. Does the doctor expect the tumour to go, or just to reduce in size? What are the chances of either happening?
7. What are the risks in having the treatment?
8. What are the short and long-term side effects during and after the treatment?
9. What diet and other alternative therapies does your doctor recommend to help minimise the side effects?

Q46. How do I best recover from chemotherapy?

As we have seen, chemotherapy works rather like radiotherapy in that it tries to kill off rapidly dividing cancer cells by poisoning them with an excess of free radicals. Unfortunately these free radicals can cause you a lot of damage. The problem with trying to define a recovery programme is that specific drugs might cause specific problems or require specific solutions to return your system back to health. Most of the general recommendations to answer this question are common to Q 41.

Whilst the chemotherapy is going on you should drink up to 3 litres of water, eat as nourishingly as you can, avoiding fats where possible, (a carbohydrate based diet is best), and consider taking 400 IU vitamin E, 200 mcgs selenium, 3000 mgs of astragalus and 2 gms soya isoflavones to help the effectiveness of the treatment. You should avoid all alcohol as your liver certainly needs no more toxins at the moment, and take milk thistle (*Silybum marianum*) (200 mgs) and soya lecithin to help to 'de-fat' it and strengthen it.

When the chemotherapy has finished, its action may well continue for weeks, and you should ask your doctor about this. There are so many different chemotherapy drugs it is impossible to generalise.

However, you need to rebuild your immune and energy systems as fast as possible. For example:

- Get a cranial osteopath to rebalance your energy and think about going to see an acupuncturist. Take a simple detox for about three days to try and clean up your system and ease back into vitamin C (4 x 500 gms) and beta-carotene (2 x 6 mgs) plus CoQ10 (30 mgs).
- Throughout the whole chemotherapy period take zinc (25 mgs) and cod liver oil (1,000 mgs) and a colloidal multivitamin and mineral supplement with good levels of vitamin B and folic acid. If the multivitamin contained iron it might be a benefit. Firstly, iron actually seems to enhance the activity of the free

radicals and so it might help the chemotherapy. Secondly, it will help boost the blood count, which has taken a hammering.

- Astragalus, cat's claw, echinacea and Essiac arc all mentioned elsewhere and may be taken after chemotherapy to re-stimulate the immune system.
- People over 35 may take wild yam to boost their DHEA levels, and eat salads and carbohydrate in the evening (carbohydrates and salads aid seratonin production, which in turn stimulates melatonin levels). Older people might even think about taking a small dose of melatonin supplement if their doctor agrees, or ornithine and argenine to stimulate Hgh.
- As with radiotherapy, you must also stimulate your body and mind.

Remember. It is a proven fact that visualisation, yoga and meditation all help boost the immune system and have a significant effect on long-term survival rates.

Fatigue

Fatigue comes free with every chemotherapy treatment. The usual recommendation is to surrender and rest.

However, research by Italian scientists (Graziano, Milan 2002), has identified that it is linked to loss of carnitine in the blood, as a result of the chemotherapy toxins.

In tests, albeit involving just 50 patients given a high energy drink contain levocarnitine (which is converted to carnitine in the body), 45 of the patients no longer felt fatigue within just one week of starting the drink. Talk to your doctor about this research.

SECTION V

Specific cancers and
their prevention

Introduction

In keeping with the intended 'easy to read' tone of this book, we look at the four leading cancers and their prevention (although some of the research evidence can also help if the cancer has already been diagnosed). This section will be far more comprehensively covered in a new book being launched in mid 2003, by Health Issues.

Q47. Tell me a little about prostate cancer?

Quick facts:

In a recorded conversation I asked the helpline of a key charity how to prevent prostate cancer, given that 'my father and brother had had it and I was over 50' (This was invented but would have made me high risk.)

Their answer was that I should eat more tomatoes and dietary fibre and less animal fat. And go for regular digital rectal examinations. I could have an annual PSA test.

They could have told me the following:

The key problem in the Western world is that every man over 50 seems to have an enlarged prostate. This is mainly due to our diet and an excess of animal fats and oestrogen in our bodies. The symptoms of an enlarged prostate and prostate cancer are extremely similar (frequency of urination, unempty bladder, etc).

A digital rectal examination will only tell you that you have an enlarged prostate. You will be sent for a PSA test if enlargement is found. A high PSA reading indicates cancer, but drinking milk or taking exercise, for example, before the test can artificially increase the reading. Even scans may be sightly misleading.

A biopsy may be taken but this is a very serious operation and may itself result in impotency and infection.

The great majority of prostate cancers are very slow growing and can be left for 10 years or more. A leading UK charity has confirmed this. Indeed the leading US charity has stated that as many as two thirds of prostate operations are probably unnecessary.

The hardest challenge for doctors is to decide whether the prostate cancer is slow growing or fast growing. In some cases even very small cancers can be fast growing and a new test for this is being developed in the UK, measuring proteins from cancer cells. As yet trials are imperfect.

Given the serious possible side effects from both operations and chemical treatments, prostate treatment should never be rushed into. This is the advice of both UK and US charities. Some things you can do to help prevent prostate cancer are:

a) Eat tomatoes (lycopene). Harvard have concluded that 7–10 helpings (especially cooked) per week reduces risk by 40 per cent, and reduces symptoms by the same amount. Lycopene reduces circulating fats in blood and displaces toxic nickel from the prostate.

b) Take saw palmetto oil. Studies show this reduces the size of an enlarged prostate.

c) Take wild yam, a natural source of progesterone which can displace and reduce levels of oestrogen in the body.

d) Lose weight; overweight men have higher oestrogen levels.

e) Reduce consumption of red meats and all animal fats as these will increase oestrogen levels.

f) Take selenium; associated with a 40 per cent lowered risk of cancer.

g) Cut out dairy; Swedish studies show a direct correlation between increased risk of prostate and the volume of dairy consumed.

h) Increase intake of vitamin D (sunshine on the body makes vitamin D from cholesterol – the pigmentation of black people prevents this and may be a reason why black people have higher prostate risk). Fish oils are a good source (but not cod liver oil).

The Mayo Clinic in 2000 and original work on eciosanoids in 1977 shows that both taking omega 3 and aspirin (81 mgs only) daily can reduce risk by 40 per cent.

In a very few cases prostate cancer can be brought on by the herpes virus. Risk is greater amongst smokers who have increased rates of vitually all cancers.

Q48. Tell me a little about breast cancer?

Quick facts

Breast cancer is largely due to one factor. Excess oestrogen. It increases the density of breast tissue and dense breast tissue is risky breast tissue.

One in eight women in the Western world will get breast cancer. This figure increases to one in six for women who take HRT, or have ever taken the pill. It becomes one in five if the pill was taken into the 30s, one in four if you smoked between the ages of 15 and 20, and one in three if you took the pill into your 40s.

Overweight women seriously increase their risk of breast cancer as do women that over-eat. Animal fats and carbohydrates in excess both stimulate oestrogen production as does regular alcohol consumption.

Refined salt and sugar consumption can increase oestrogen levels through their influence on other hormone levels such as insulin.

Dairy consumption is a very big negative influence, whilst soy, or soya, consumption is a positive influence. The recent research study in Singapore by three top cancer bodies seals this view. Phytooestrogens from soy, red clover and pulses like chickpeas, although weaker in their effect than human oestrogen, are sufficiently similar in biochemical structure to be able to bind to receptor sites on healthy cells whilst having no carcinogenic effect. This action blocks the receptors from accepting normal oestrogen which causes the stimulation of breast cancer.

A bigger picture has to be looked at when considering breast cancer.

Centuries ago women had less periods, because of lifestyle and dietary factors. Periods occurred between the ages of 18–38, and more babies and breast feeding periods of up to two years cut the number of monthly oestrogen bursts from today's levels of around 440 per lifetime to around 240.

Higher consumption of animal fats and alcohol, aided and abetted by smoking, worsens this. Significantly lower levels of vegetable, fruit, and pulse consumption provides less protection, whilst high levels of dairy consumption in the West are clearly implicated.

Some breast cancer appears linked to the herpes virus after exposure to chicken pox or shingles.

But the problems do not stop there for women.

Recycled water in cities contains oestrogen residues, and they are constantly exposed to oestrogen mimics in the environment, for example, volatile organic carbon compounds leaching from carpets to computers, from cleaning agents to furniture polish, from breathing petrol fumes to certain perfumes on the skin.

Neither self-examination nor mammograms have been conclusively shown to reduce death rates from the disease, in fact it is arguable that mammograms can actually worsen the overall risk of breast cancer. Research in the USA in 2002 cast serious doubt on even the validity of their results.

What is a girl to do?

a) Well if you don't want more children, you could certainly breast feed them longer. Not least of all because breast fed children have less illness and higher IQs!

b) Cut dairy, ideally completely.

c) Cut animal fats and excess carbohydrates.

d) Do not be overweight.

e) Do not smoke, never take the pill or HRT.

f) Take wild yam or use natural progesterone creams.

g) Use glass bottled water, or a reverse osmosis filter for all water supplies (including cooking and hot drinks).

h) Eat more fresh vegetables and fruit. More soy and pulses. Women with the highest consumption of soya have less breast cancer (Cancer Research UK/Sloan Kettering).

i) Eat more garlic – found in the Iowa study to reduce cancer in women.

j) Take tocopherol vitamin E. (In European countries only tocophenol is licensed for sale.) Found in palm oil this collects in breast tissue and reduces its density.

k) As does vitamin A and omega 3. In fact women with the highest levels of omega 3 in their circulation have no breast cancer.

l) Eat organic and fresh. Pesticides and some preservatives increase oestrogen levels.

Some women will be identified as higher risk; women who have a mother or sister with the disease. They can also be identified with certain genes.

BRCA1 damage allows cancer cells to hide from immune system searching cells.

BRCA2 damage prevents the normal repair of DNA damage.

Medical opinion is that these women should have mastectomies or take preventative tamoxifen. Tamoxifen like all chemical agents can have an effect although this can be limited and side-effects, including other cancers, may occur.

Women in the highest risk categories need to take the highest care of themselves. General antioxidant boosters and cancer preventative measures should be employed. Prevention is the key.

Finally high doses of vitamin C have been shown to be especially effective in the prevention of breast cancer *and* in extending life expectancy of those already diagnosed.

ERRATUM
Pg 200 point J should read
Take Tocotrienol Vitamin E (In European countries only Tocopherol is licensed for sale).

Q49. Tell me a little about lung cancer?

Quick facts

There is some 'hereditary' link where lung cancer is concerned but this is more likely to be an hereditary link to cancer in general.

Women have a greater risk of smoking-induced lung cancer than men because they have two X chromosomes whilst men have only one. This doubles factors, found in the airways, that link to levels of lung cancer.

Smoking causes increased risk of lung cancer, it is a proven fact. With lowered incidence of smoking in Britain, lung cancers are in decline, and by 2005 may well have fallen to third behind prostate an breast cancer incidence.

However other causes are radon and diesel fumes. Indeed, smoking coupled with radon or diesel fumes has been shown to considerably amplify the risks.

A few lung cancers may be caused by X-rays or occur a number of years after radiotherapy on breast tissue.

Clearly to prevent lung cancer:

a) Avoid smoking.
b) Avoid smoke filled places and people who smoke.
c) Have your house checked for radon. Carpets worsen levels of dust in the air as do closed windows and doors.
d) Avoid living in cities or next to main roads.

Other general cancer preventative steps like taking antioxidants pale into insignificance behind the above factors.

Q50. Tell me a little about colon cancer?

Quick facts

Colon cancer risk can be hereditary but there is much you can do to prevent this cancer.

The UK charity provides the followig advice:
- Cut animal fats and red meat
- Cut alcohol consumption
- Eat more vegetables and fibre
- Cut caffeine consumption
- Watch your weight
- Increase fluid intake and watch your bowel movements!

This is by no means all you can do. Research indicates the following:

a) In the Iowa study there was a clear link between garlic consumption and reduced levels of colon cancer.

b) Both animal fats and alcohol increase the production of a carcinogenic bile acid. Consuming these two 'foods' literally causes you to poison yourself. Omega 3 and vitamin D cause suppression of this acid. (Fish oils – but not natural cod liver oil unless supplemented – provide both.)

c) Aspirin in small doses also has this effect, whilst furthermore it reduces the size of pre-cancerous polyps.

d) Folic acid has been clearly shown to reduce colon and bowel cancer.

e) Taking acidophilus and other friendly bacteria is no bad thing.

f) Finally, everybody over 50 (but particularly men) can be annually screened. Sigmoidoscopy seems to be the favoured and safe method.

Increase your antioxidant levels, keep a clean liver, avoiding parasites, maintain regular soft bowel movements, take in plenty of clean water and fresh vegetables. Follow the general principles of cancer prevention.

SECTION VI

You really can beat cancer

A summary

Introduction

If you want to beat cancer and you live in the West you need to be radical, disciplined and dedicate some serious time, effort and love to yourself. You must create your own micro-environment within a world that is increasingly full of dangers and attempt to reverse the surrounding trend of worsening odds, for yourself and those you love. You must start by reviewing your whole life.

Here are the five key principles:

Your diet

o *Get back to basics with simple fresh foods and base your diet around fruit, vegetables and whole brown rice*
o *Cut out the 'bad guys' (especially smoking, alcohol, sugar and caffeine) and introduce the good guys (see diet page)*
o *Supplement, detox and cleanse parasites and yeasts.*

Your lifestyle

o *Exercise daily; think slim*
o *Take up t'ai chi and/or yoga*
o *Go for three monthly body energy checks*
o *Cut the problems out of your life, or at least manage them better*
o *Reduce the risks of catching viruses.*

Your environment

o *Review all your household, cosmetic and toiletry products*
o *Avoid all radiation and magnetic fields*
o *Avoid all drugs whenever possible*
o *Avoid strong sunlight.*

Your mind

o *Learn to meditate*
o *List your strengths; develop your self-worth and self-esteem*
o *Take time for yourself*
o *Develop a plan for the future and a sense of purpose.*

Your soul

o *Think about your place in the Universe, now and in the future. Think about religion*
o *Practise acts of kindness, be friendly, helpful, look for strengths in others, use your own.*

Summary 1.

How to beat cancer:
the 30 point checklist for everybody

1. Avoid all fats and oils, especially animal fats, and fats and oils in cooking. Use olive oil if you need to, but in moderation.
2. Do not smoke.
3. Reduce alcohol intake to two to three glasses of Cabernet Sauvignon per week.
4. Do not be overweight. Ideally be 5 per cent underweight for your height.
5. Eat nourishingly. Consume more carbohydrate and less animal protein. Consume more vegetables, fruits and rice, plus beans, pulses, garlic and ginger. Think vegetables and fruit first. Have three meat-free days per week.
6. Ideally consume slightly less calories than you need per day. Eat six small meals rather than three big ones.
7. Eat raw, steamed, roasted but not microwaved, fried or barbecued food.
8. Juice fresh fruits and vegetables yourself
9. Drink soya milk, eat soya products. Try to avoid dairy, even small amounts; beware hidden dairy in cakes and biscuits, for example.
10. Don't drink fizzy soft drinks, especially low calorie ones
11. Avoid sugar, salt and caffeine. Drink green tea. Beware hidden salt and sugar in breakfast cereals or processed foods and remember mass produced juices are big sources of sugar.
12. Remove products which contain carcinogens from your everyday life.
13. Avoid electromagnetic radiation, near the house or in the bedroom. Beware mobile phones and radon.
14. Avoid all drugs where possible; avoid antibiotics
15. Be monogamous.
16. Women should avoid extra oestrogen eg the pill or HRT

17. Check regularly (once a year) for virus or parasite problems; keep yeasts at bay; take acidophilus.
18. Take cod liver oil every day.
19. Take supplements, especially the magnificent six. Have short periods during the year when you boost your herbal intake, especially astragalus, Essiac and echinacea, particularly if you've been unwell.
20. Drink filtered water from glass bottles.
21. Spend one hour a day looking after yourself.
22. Take some exercise daily. Try to exercise for seven hours a week. Do some resistance training.
23. Have a body energy service regularly, for example, every three months, with a cranial osteopath and/or an acupuncturist.
24. Love your lymph and move it daily with yoga exercises or some t'ai chi.
25. Calm yourself, free your brain, learn to relax, learn to meditate.
26. Learn about yourself, write a checklist of the things (including people) that limit you and avoid them. Don't put up with things that make you unhappy or depressed. Never feel guilty, subservient, desperate to please others or indebted. See friends, go to the gym, see a counsellor and/or doctor. Concentrate on the things that you enjoy and are your skills.
27. Establish your sense of purpose. What do you really want to be doing in three years or with the rest of your life? Write it down and stick it on the bathroom wall so you read it every morning. Remember. You can do it, or you can make excuses.
28. Discover your own spirituality. Think about how you interact with others; your body energy, inside and outside of you; think about how it interacts with the universe. Consider God and a religion. Practise acts of kindness, be helpful and understanding.
29. Fill your days with happiness and real value. Keep moving forward, don't live in the past.
30. Celebrate life.

Summary 2.

Supplements:
the checklist for non-sufferers ←

Remember, nothing beats the real foods as they will always contain many more active ingredients. The following is a list of products with which to supplement your diet each day, if you are not on other medication or undergoing chemotherapy or radio-therapy. Here are my personal suggestions:

Beta-carotene	6–12 mgs (take during the day eg 3 x 4 mgs or 2 x 6 mgs)
Vitamin C	1 gm time-released (including rosehips/bioflavonoids)
Vitamin E	400 IU (286 mgs)
Zinc	15–25 mgs
Selenium	50–150 mcgs (max 200 mcgs)
CoQ10	30 mgs
Soya lecithin	3 gms max
Soya isoflavones	2 gms max
Garlic tablets	2–3 x 600 mgs tablets (equivalent to 500 gm of fresh clove)
Cod liver oil or fish oils	1,000 mgs

Doses given are for adults only. For children please consult your physician. People under 20 should not take CoQ10. Do not take vitamin C if you have been diagnosed with a primary or secondary brain tumour.

Plus a good multivitamin and multimineral supplement (ideally colloidal) that contains B vitamins and folic acid (400 mcgs) plus traces of a wide range of minerals and amino acids.

Men can also take lycopene (10–20 mgs) and saw palmetto (400 mgs)

Consider eating apricot kernels (5–10 a day) and taking astra-galus, echinacea and Essiac, especially if you've been unwell.

And if you don't eat much fruit, drink Noni juice. The EU has currently banned its sale in Europe as it is a speciality food, and to date, there is no maximum safe consumption level set. Recent reports suggest it will return to sale soon.

Summary 3.

The action checklist for the cancer sufferer

NB This assumes a programme of surgery, then radiotherapy, then chemotherapy. See section IV for more details.

Phase A   Diagnosis

1. Get a 'buddy'.
2. Develop a plan with your doctor and your 'buddy'. Try to work out what caused your cancer and what might be sustaining it.
3. Check everything you are told; get a second opinion, go on the internet. Demand answers.
4. Go for a virus, parasite and yeast check.
5. Cut out all possible carcinogens from your world immediately:

   - smoking, alcohol, caffeine, the pill, HRT
   - sugar, salt, preservatives, dried/smoked meats, crisps and snack foods
   - all dairy (including live yoghurt)
   - all refined and processed foods
   - all fried foods, all fats and oils, except olive oil
   - all red meats, farmed meats and farmed fish; go organic
   - your mobile phone, cordless phone, take the TV from the bedroom, don't sleep between lights
   - clear your house and garden of toxins

6. Start taking gentle exercise every day, if you've done none before. Go to a yoga class, learn to meditate. In 10 weeks going three times per week you'll be good enough!
7. Find a cranial osteopath, acupuncturist, homeopath and visualiser all of whom have experience dealing with cancer and ideally your sort.
8. Buy a three to ten day detox. Take daily, to help your liver

   - 200 mgs milk-thistle (*Silybum marianum*)
   - 3 gms soya lecithin

9. Use the diet plan in the book and add in the following supplements:
   - Cod liver oil   1,000 mgs per day
   - Beta-carotene   2–3 x 6 mgs per day at intervals
   - Vitamin C   1–3 x 1 gm per day at intervals
   - Vitamin E   400–1,000 IU per day
   - Zinc   1–3 x 15 mgs
   - Selenium   200 mcgs
   - Coenzyme Q10   30 mgs per day (especially if you are over 50)
   - Lycopene   15–25 mgs
   - 2 x 2 Garlic tablets per day
   - A colloidal multivitamin, mineral and amino acid supplement (preferably containing no iron).

   Doses given are for adults only. For children please consult your physician. Do not take vitamin C if you have been diagnosed with a primary or secondary brain tumour. People under 20 should not take CoQ10. Some supplements should not be taken during radiotherapy treatment, see page 215.

10. Change to soya milk, and take 3 gms soya isoflavones per day.
11. Change to green tea, Essiac and drink at least 1.5 litres of water per day. Take astragalus and echinacea.
12. Consider taking Noni juice and apricot kernels. Use the list of alkaline producing foods. Eat garlic and ginger; take acidophilus.
13. Take linusit (2 tablespoons) with breakfast; or psyllium pills.

It is a lot to take but you need to boost your defences as quickly and as effectively as possible.

Phase B   Surgery

14. Keep with the plan above plus
    - buy vitamin E cream to reduce scars
    - think about talking with a homeopath to aid recovery

Phase C   Radiotherapy approaching
15. Detox three to five days
16. Buy aloe vera gel to put on target area.

Phase D   During radiotherapy and after for four to six weeks
17. Go with someone to every session. Do not miss a session.
18. Take the supplements previously listed **especially** selenium and soya isoflavones and astragalus.

19. But do <u>not</u> take any
  – Vitamin C
  – Beta-carotene
  – Lycopene
  – Coenzyme Q10
  – Essiac

And cut the vitamin E to 400 IU.

20. The multivitamin and multimineral may now contain iron.
21. Eat lots of organic eggs and raw garlic. Take kelp supplements and extra folic acid (in total about 800 mcgs – there were 400 mcgs in the multivitamin). All of this will help your hair stay in place and help protect your good DNA.
22. Increase water intake to 3 litres per day.
23. Keep up the yoga if possible; and especially the meditation and visualisation. You should stop reiki, cranial osteopathy and acupuncture during this time.

Phase E   After the radiotherapy has ceased to work
24. Talk to the doctor about your progress; get other opinions.
25. Get back to exercise and yoga. See the cranial osteopath, acupuncturist, healer and homeopath again, and get another programme sorted out.
26. Start taking the vitamin C, beta-carotene, lycopene and coenzyme Q10 again as in Phase A.

27. Keep with the plan for diet and supplements in Phase A
    Definitely take:

    - Echinacea
    - Astralagus
    - Cat's claw
    - Wild yam
      (take the amounts indicated on the bottle).

28. Keep any yeasts and parasites at bay
29. Take some organic iron for seven days to boost your blood
    count.

Phase F   Chemotherapy

NB The run up to chemotherapy, the course and then the activity afterwards are more dependent upon the actual drug used, so you must consult your doctor.

30. Check any proposed drug on the internet. Get a second
    opinion
31. By and large repeat the radiotherapy plan.

Phase G   Establishing your new life

32. Remember all those promises you made to yourself.......
    'When I get better, I'm going to ...?' Stick to your new life
    plan, your new diet, your new activities. Keep the bad
    things out of your life. New goals, new sense of purpose. Be
    happy with who you are, not who you think others want
    you to be
33. Celebrate life.

Don't eat	Do eat
Any farmed meat; red meat	Free range chickens, ducks, game
Any farmed fish, prawns, coastal fish	Deep sea caught fish
Any dried meats, cooked meats or sausages, smoked meats or fish	Have vegetarian days – two or three days a week
Any dairy, milk, cheese, margarine, yoghurts	All soya, tofu, tempeh, miso, soya sauce (Shoyu & Tamari)
Live yoghurt	Acidophilus
Ice cream	Sorbet
Dips	Hummous in olive oil
Fast food	The fish from fish & chips (if you have to)
Refined wheat, flour, sugar & salt; processed foods, chips, junk food	Oats, buckwheat, millet, organic brown rice (complete), fresh foods
Wheat, breakfast cereals, muesli	Home made cereal
Crisps, peanuts	Pumpkin/sunflower & sesame seeds, organic dried fruits
Chocolate, coffee, tea	Home made lemon & ginger & honey; Cassie tea green tea with lemon grass
Cakes, biscuits, white bread	10 helpings of fruit and vegatables per day
E numbers	Garlic, chives, onions and leeks
Oranges, lemons, rhubarb, tomatoes (don't eat too many)	Bean sprouts, alfalfa, fennel, grilled tomatoes
Tap water in plastic bottles	Filtered boiled water. Glass bottled water
Barbecued or boiled or fried or microwaved food	Steam, roast, stew if you can't eat raw!
Gelatine	Agar-agar

Diet plan checklist

hy?
rmed meat contains added hormones, antibiotics and pesticides from fields; cook well to stroy natural hormones.
rmed fish (most prawns and salmon are farmed) again contains antibiotics and colorants. astal fish contain many toxins. Deep sea oily fish that has been caught is excellent (when ing out).
ied meats and sausages again can contain antibiotics and added growth hormones, but also servatives and nitrites.
lk (even goat's milk) contains hormones, antibiotics and pesticides. IGF-1 from milk directly ked to cancers in prostate and breast. Soya contains active cancer blockers.
iry as above
iry as above
ickpeas contain isoflavones which block tumours.
t food is often cooked in hydrogenated vegetable oil which spreads free radicals, hits the nune system and makes bad eicosanoids.
cessed food, sugar & salt weaken the immune system. Should eat organic whole brown each day; eat fresh foods, nourishing foods and build your body energy.
inkle linseeds (Linusit), millet bran, pumpkin seeds, sunflower & sesame seeds over oats breakfast. Use Soya milk and honey to sweeten.
drogenated oils, salt, preservatives & colouring replaced by organic natural sources of min E & isoflavones. Crisps, chips, cereals, biscuits contain acrylamides.
ocolate, coffee, tea are no-go areas. Green tea with lemon grass is a real antioxidant ture, as is Cassie tea or: pour hot water onto slices of fresh lemon and ginger with a little ey.
es, biscuits contain fats & milk. White bread is refined and full of salt, sugar & preserva- s. Beware brown bread – look for *wholegrain, wholemeal*. Try lemon grass, Brussels outs, cabbage, broccoli, kale, apricots, peaches, pineapples and papaya (red & yellow ts and veg). Salads of avocados, red and yellow peppers, watercress, herbs, carrots.
not overcook or you will lose the anti-cancer agents allicin, selenium, germanium, stine.
se fruits are good in moderation but very acid. Try juicing watercress & fennel or green les (organic without wax or preservatives). Alfalfa is highly nutritious, as are bean outs.
d parasites and nasty minerals. Avoid toxins from plastic bottles; filter your own water.
ng raw vegetables before meal gives you 40 per cent more vitamins; fried gives you bad overboiling takes away vitamins; barbecued makes carcinogens (nitrosamines).
p the animal fat out of your cooking.

THE POSTSCRIPT

Catherine's 'Survival'

The 31 August 2001 was Catherine's 23rd birthday. The evening before, she was given her first 'all clear'. One presumes that this is what is termed 'remission', but they used no such couched jargon, simply the words all clear. The MRI scan showed the scar tissue from her operation, a large number of dead cancer cells but none that were living or growing.

Three months later another scan still failed to find any cancer cells, as did another in May 2002. One eminent surgeon following the case described this as most definitely a miracle. Apparently he had been told things were pretty hopeless and that she had less than six months to live back in May 2001. No one said anything like this to us at the time, but whatever we thought or feared was anyway lost under a mountain of determination, teamwork and effort.

Perhaps I should provide a little more information and detail.

When Catherine was told she needed surgery, we urgently put her on 1 gm of time-released vitamin C a day, 1,000 mgs of cod liver oil, 1,000 IU of vitamin E and 30 mgs zinc. This little cocktail and Mr Kitchen's excellent work with the knife are responsible for almost negligible scarring despite a cut from the centre of her crown to below her ear just in front of the hairline.

But there was more. Fearing the worst from day one, two weeks before anyone mentioned the dreaded 'C' word, we added to the above, 15 mgs beta-carotene, 200 mcgs of selenium, plus Neway's Maximol, a quality colloidal multivitamin with minerals and amino acids, 15 mgs lycopene and 30 mgs Coenzyme Q10 simply to boost her immune system on a daily basis.

By the time the worst was confirmed we had received some serious supplies of supplements and also had a theory for how her illness had come about.

No-one in the medical profession seemed bothered about what had caused Catherine's brain tumour. Catherine ate no fruit, she used a mobile phone to the tune of £150 plus per month, was on the pill and drank to excess like most other female students. I must admit I was shocked when I found out she also smoked up to 25 cigarettes a day. She talked a good exercise class but I doubt she participated too often, and she also had a fairly typical cancer sufferer's psychological profile. She liked to please everyone else, put herself bottom of the list, did things for peer group approval and often felt guilty about letting people down when she clearly hadn't. Catherine certainly had the odds stacked against her.

There was however another factor that worried me. In her first 18 months of university (about three years previously) she had had tonsillitis frequently. She had had this illness all her life, but only once a year. At university she was having it every six weeks. The doctors were prescribing the usual amoxycillin and she would take Ibuprofen.

Then I read an article about yeasts and how if you take lots of antibiotics it killed the good bacteria in your stomach, allowing the yeasts to come out to play. So two years ago she started taking caprylic acid, oregano, garlic and Pau d'Arco, with a ban on wheat (previously her favourite foods were pasta, bread and pizza) for the summer. The result was that she recovered and had 10 months tonsillitis-free. When it did recur she went to a cranial osteopath who said that my solution was pretty well right but gave her a longer list of ingredients to avoid, and moved her body energy around as it was concentrated in her overactive stomach area, with none around her head and neck. The result. No more tonsillitis.

However I now believe that greater effects were already taking place in her body.

Yeasts are notorious weakeners of the immune system, which is one reason the tonsillitis continually reappeared. They drain the body of all vitamins, particularly B vitamins. Catherine's lifestyle of tobacco, alcohol, stress, lack of sleep and the pill would have seen off any vitamin B that did actually make it past the yeasts.

But B complex vitamins include three components essential to DNA and the brain. Folic acid is essential for the accurate replication of DNA in dividing cells. Choline and inositol are rare in that they can pass through the blood/brain barrier and they are known to nourish the brain cells.

Worse, in the American book 'Brain Fitness' the two authors Dr Klatz and Dr Goldman describe antibiotics and anti-inflammatories as two of their six 'brain poisons' and antibiotics are known to prevent proper absorption of folic acid. All this was building up a picture of why she may have had had this failure in her left frontal lobe. (I should add that if mobile phones were linked to brain tumours, experts believe they would more likely appear at the side of the head.) Another possible cause, Aspartame, is being studied in research in the UK right now but I had told the children my fears about Aspartame four years before and they had ceased drinking diet drinks.

Rather like Dr Jane Plant in her book, my view was, 'If we can work out a likely cause, we can also work out what is sustaining the cancer and act upon that.'

My theory led me to write a diet for Catherine, a modified and more general version of which appears in this book. My principles for Catherine were:

- kill off the yeasts and any parasites
- return a good supply of Vitamin B especially to the brain
- remove all antibiotics from the diet
- cut all the toxins out of her life
- give her an alkaline body
- rebuild her immune system and strenthen her for the inevitable radiotherapy.

The anti-yeast programme meant removing all wheat from the diet, stopping all alcohol, eating no mushrooms, marrow's, courgettes, melons, cucumber, fruit juices and fruits (easy for Catherine) and taking caprylic acid, Pau d'Arco, garlic, Echinacea and acidophilus.

For a multivitamin and mineral supplement she took four units of Neway's Maximol, colloidal liquid per day. This had several benefits. Catherine was taking enough pills already and it was a liquid; the list of contents was amazingly comprehensive covering amino acids as well as minerals and vitamins; it contained fulvate/fulvic acid which is the naturally occurring active ingredient in plant roots that enables minerals to pass more easily from the soil into the plant; and finally it is a colloidal *suspension of a type known to be easily absorbed.*

It is worth adding here that I do not believe that much of a vitamin pill is actually absorbed by the body. Some estimates show this figure to be as low as 20 per cent (this is why most of her supplements were in a natural organic form). With a colloid I felt Catherine would really charge her system quickly. I did however add a B complex every two days for its folic acid content and gave her soya lecithin (for inositol and choline) and soya isoflavones.

As antioxidants we gave her 400 IU of vitamin E, 1 gm of vitamin C (time release) and 2 x 6 mgs beta-carotene. She was also taking 200 mcgs selenium and coenzyme Q10 30mgs and 25 mgs lycopene.

She took 1,000 mgs of cod liver oil every two days to try and reduce and replace her 'bad fats' content with omega 3 and enhance her vitamin A levels to fight the cancer.

Her diet was changed to reflect all this with much more fresh garlic, olive oil, salads and fish. We bought her lemongrass and galanga, green teas and Essiac, replaced all the milk with soya and she cut out caffeine and sugar.

She was given a bowl containing pumpkin seeds and sunflower seeds to munch instead of crisps. And chocolate, tea, coffee and dairy were banned. Her consumption of water rose markedly and she took Neway's Noni juice as I was very worried about her lack of fruit consumption and the likelihood of her body being on the acid side of the desired pH line.

When Catherine started her radiotherapy four weeks later she came off all the beta-carotene, vitamin C, lycopene and coenzyme Q10, any of which could have lessened the desired effect of the radiation.

As I was concerned about the possibility of parasites linked to cancer, she also took an anti-parasite product, Neway's purge.

Yes, she was taking a lot of supplements but we were in an urgent and corrective situation.

Her radiotherapy lasted six weeks, she went to every session and someone always went with her for mental and moral support.

By now she was tired and had lost her hair. Some days her depression was so evident you could have weighed it.

During the last two weeks of radiotherapy we talked a lot. We stayed together in London and went to the tennis at Wimbledon, saw 'Mamma Mia', and 'Chicago' and we did fun things. We talked through an idea to produce a regular magazine for doctors and patients alike on all the latest developments in cancer; be it about clinical trials on drugs in Boston or successful case histories on visualisation techniques at Bristol.

I had been busy trying to track down a supplier of B-17 but had run up against the FDA bans. But a friend who had spare apricot kernels – her sister in America was sending them for their mother's cancer (with great success I must add) – provided a pack of those. This, if nothing else, saved my mother from eating apricots and banging the stones open with a hammer in the back garden every day! From about week four of the radiotherapy Catherine started to eat 30 kernels a day and take bromelain and papain supplements (Oh, that she would eat pineapple or papaya!).

When the radiotherapy finished, we went to my house in France for a month with her sisters and brother and a selection of girl friends, and had some fun and fresh air. We used the time to refocus Catherine on her future happiness, lifestyle and sense of purpose. I couldn't stop Catherine drinking Rosé, but on top of her normal supplements we reintroduced beta-carotene (2 x 6 mgs) but this time in the form of Neway's Cascading Revenol which has beta-carotene and a mix of other antioxidants, plus astralagus, cat's claw, wild yam, lycopene and organic iron (the latter just for one week) all to rebuild her immune system and her blood count as fast as possible. I just used to hand her different pills at different times of the day so I'm not even sure she knew what she was taking. Except that it was a lot.

I had finally managed to get hold of some B-17, having chased round the internet. Catherine took 6,500 mgs tablets a day, plus 6 tablets of Megazyme, a mixture of bromelain, papain, pancreatic enzymes and other helpful ingredients. She did, however, use the B-17 pills as an excuse to give up the apricot kernels, which were too bitter for her liking.

Interestingly when she saw her oncologist for a routine update meeting, he blamed her heartburn on 'the B-17 turning to hydrogen cyanide in her stomach'. It doesn't.

Catherine has also refocused her lifestyle. The smoking, the pill and most of the dairy consumption have gone. She goes to the gym very regularly and attends three yoga classes a week. Her weight (she was never particularly overweight) has tumbled from the steroid induced size of Autumn 2001. She is back at work full-time and has had a full, successful and productive 2002.

Who knows what worked in this cocktail of radiotherapy, fun and supplements? Do I care? Well, yes actually I do. I genuinely wish I could say it was a combination of these two or three things so that others could really benefit from our knowledge. All I can say is, 'Somewhere in this mix, a combination of factors seemed to deliver a result and ....so far, so good'.

Catherine has recently had her fourth all clear and doesn't have to go back for a check up for at least six months, maybe a year.

A malignant brain tumour is with you always. It is very dangerous. Fingers crossed!

And Next?

I am convinced that across the hundreds of books written and the wealth of information on the internet, the solutions for cancer are already known; but some heads will have to be banged together to encourage a more genuine belief in this by the people officially in charge of our country's health. The medical profession has no exclusive mandate on curing cancer but sadly they are almost exclusively the focus of funding from the Government, drug companies and sponsors. It is hard to see how one oncologist could understand the full benefits of meditation or how a sense of purpose filters down from the brain to alter the biochemistry of a prostate cell. It is simply too big a subject for any one person to become a complete expert in.

At some point the status quo must change to provide genuine through the line teamwork that brings all the possible solutions together into a managed package for sufferers. Shouldn't every hospital cancer unit offer 'complementary help'? Shouldn't every hospital try to give you a personal manager who can help you get the best out of all the known treatments, be they radiotherapy or visualisation, vitamin supplementation, or analysis of possible causes?

Laurens Van der Post began a campaign in 1982 aimed at persuading the medical establishment to form closer ties with complementary practitioners. In 1998 the NHS approved £18.4m to renovate the Royal London Homeopathic Hospital, its 'principal complementary medicine provider' and in 2001 there were reports of the Prince of Wales backing Dr Mosaref Ali to form his integrated hospital. I am pleased to note Macmillan's recent directory of 300 complementary services in the UK, of which approximately one third are attached to hospitals and hospices. These are but small steps in the right direction.

But my personal view is that the Government should pledge a large sum of money for the next 50 years to finance an independent body to review, and have the power to tackle, prevention issues. This should be independent of the medical profession, the Government, the health service and the drugs companies. The body should be allowed to have real control and to properly use the law and even change it when, for example, it sees toxins being used in everyday products or produced by factories, it wants hard facts on the long term effect of pesticides or GM foods, or it feels there are health considerations on electromagnetic fields which should over-rule current planning approvals on pylons and transmitters by local authorities on largely aesthetic grounds. It would be a massive undertaking and one that might take time to bring results even if the will were there, but it is absolutely essential to the health of the nation.

We need a body that is the people's champion and doesn't have the slightest hint of any relationship with any one with any interest, other than the genuine desire to reduce the levels of cancer contracted in the future.

Having spent the last two years immersed in this vast and complex world of cancer, I am convinced it can be beaten and the truth is we probably know enough already to do it. But the route we are taking now simply cannot be right for either us or our children.

Chris Woollams
February 2003

APPENDICES

APPENDIX I

Acid Residue Producers - a fuller list

FRUITS

- Bananas
- Grapefruit
- Oranges
- Plums
- Prunes

VEGETABLES

- Asparagus tips
- Brussel sprouts
- Chick peas
- Dried beans
- Lentils
- Peanuts
- Rhubarb
- Tomatoes

ALL DAIRY

ALL FLESH FOODS

- Meats, fish, shellfish, scallops, crab,
- All processed and salted meats, smoked fish

CEREALS AND NUTS

- All packet nuts, crisps and snacks
- All refined flour including noodles, spaghetti, buckwheat
- Barley
- Cornflakes and most processed breakfast cereals
- Doughnuts
- Dumplings
- Macaroni
- Oatmeal
- Pies, pastries and bread
- Refined rice

OTHER

- All alcohol
- Chocolate, cocoa
- Coffee, tea
- Fizzy drinks
- Eggs
- Lack of sleep
- Negative emotions
- Preservatives, jams etc
- Products in vinegar
- Salt & condiments
- Sauces
- Stress
- Sugar
- Sweets
- Tobacco
- Vinegar

Alkaline Residue Products - a fuller list

FRESH FRUITS
Apple
Apricot
Avocado
Blackberries
Blackcurrants
Cherries
Cranberries
Currants, raisins
Dates
Figs
Grapes
Lemons
Lychees
Mangoes
Melon
Olives
Papaya
Peach
Pear
Raspberries
Redcurrants

OTHER
Alfalfa
Agar-Agar
Fresh cracked nuts
Fresh ginger
Fresh juices (own preparation)
Herb teas, green tea
Honey
Millet
Noni juice
Olive oil, corn oil
Seeds
Soya products

VEGETABLES
Aubergines
Beetroot
Broccoli
Cabbage
Carrots, parsnips
Cauliflower
Celery
Chard
Chicory
Chives
Cucumber
Dandelion
Dill
Endive
Fresh green beans
Garlic
Kale
Kelp
Lettuce
Mushrooms
Parsnips
Peppers
Potatoes
Noni juice
Radishes
Sorrel
Soya beans
Spinach
Squash
Swede
Turnips
Watercress

APPENDIX II
Useful Contacts

Telephone

a) Cancer Helplines – Specific

Bladder Cancer	0207 831 9831
Brain Tumours (S D R T)	0125 261 7843
Breast Cancer Care Helpline	0808 800 6000
Colon Cancer Helpline	0207 381 4711
International Myeloma Foundation	0800 980 3332
Kidney Cancer UK	0247 647 0584
Leukaemia Research Fund	0207 269 9068
Lung Cancer (Roy Castle Foundation)	0800 357 7200
Ovarian Cancer UK	0207 600 5141
Pancreatic Cancer	0121 449 0667
Prostate Cancer Helpline	0845 300 8383

b) Cancer Helplines – Complementary & Integrated

Bristol Cancer Centre Helpline	0117 980 9500
Gerson UK	01204 593 746
The Dove Clinic	02074 865 588
The Hale Clinic	0870 167 6667
The Haven (Breast Cancer)	0207 384 0000
The Nutritional Cancer Therapy Trust	01271 850 122
The Institute for Complementary Medicines	0207 237 5165

c) Cancer Helplines – General

Cancer BACUP Helpline	0808 800 1234
Cancer Research UK	0207 269 3142
Cancerlink Helpline	0808 808 0000
Cancer Resource Centre	0207 924 3924
Macmillan Cancer Relief	0845 601 6161
Marie Curie Cancer Care	0800 716 146
The Patients Association	0208 423 8999

b) Other useful numbers

Allergy and Vitamin Testing	0238 081 2124

British Acupuncture Council	0208 735 0400
The Association of Colonic Hydrotherapists	0144 282 7687
The Society of Homeopaths	0160 462 1400
The British Federation of Massage Practitioners	0177 288 1063
The British Assn of Nutritional Therapists	0870 606 1284
Institute for Optimum Nutrition	0208 877 9993
National Radiological Protection Board	0800 614 529
The Sutherland Society (Cranial Osteopathy)	0122 5869 100

Web sites

1. General Sites

Cancer Guide
www.cancerguide.org
This site gives you info on how to find what you want and get the best possible treatments.

Cancer Bacup
www.cancerbacup.org.uk
The UK's leading information service. Very professional, regularly updated with tailor made service, publications, nurse and links to other sites. Top notch with over 100 local centres throughout the UK. Good for rare cancers.

Cancer Research UK
www.cancerresearchuk.org
Largest cancer charity in Europe with a site to match. Latest news, links to specific sites. 'Everything you need to know about cancer' (now, where have we heard that before!)

National Cancer Institute
www.nci.nih.gov
A bit formal, US site covering all cancer types with treatment information, news on latest development projects and trials. Massive.

American Cancer Society
www.cancer.org
The definitive US site; news, information, and latest developments. Easy to use.

Royal Marsden Hospital
www.royalmarsden.org
Brilliant site from UK's top cancer unit. Find out about everything jargon-free. Good information booklets, latest news.

Memorial Sloan-Kettering
www.mskcc.org
New York gold standard cancer treatment centre with information to match. Very clinical.

2. Carers, Self Help and Home Support

Macmillan Cancer relief
www.macmillan.org.uk
Support for people with cancer and their families. Aim to provide best support, treatment and care. Access to 2000 nurses for community and home help. Now joined forces with .....

Marie Curie
www.mariecurie.org.uk
Care for thousands of people in their own homes and at hospices throughout the UK.

3. Integrated and Complementary

The Bristol Cancer Help Centre
www.bristolcancerhelp.org
'We practice, teach, research and develop the holistic approach as an integral part of cancer care'. The professionals.

The Haven Trust
www.thehaventrust.org.uk
Breast cancer site with emphasis on complementary therapies, counselling, and support services.

The Dove Clinic for Integrated Medicine
www.doveclinic.com
Screening, complementary treatment and counselling in London and Winchester.

Gerson Therapy

www.gerson.org

American site offering advice on the treatment, with newsletter and books

Nutritional Cancer Therapy Trust

sarah@flower-iridol.freeserve.co.uk

UK site covering nutritional therapy and based on Dr Plaskett's revisions to, and updating of, Gerson.

4. Specific

Brain

www.sdrt.intec.co.uk

UK independent site, helpful with good research list.

Breast – Breast care

www.breastcancercare.org.uk

Free publications and booklets. Refer you to phone line. Good link to-

The Lavender Trust

www.lavendertrustfund.org.uk

Breast cancer site aimed at the problems faced by younger women, with great details on benefits and state financial assistance.

Colon

www.coloncancer.org.uk

Excellent and frequently updated site, offering news research and advice.

Leukaemia

www.leukaemia.org

(USA) Information for new patients, research, news and support systems.

Lung Cancer

www.roycastle.org.

The Roy Castle Lung Cancer Foundation is the only charity in the world dedicated to lung cancer; support groups, dedicated nurses, research, even quit smoking programs.

Melanoma
www.cancer.org.au
Australians know more about melanoma than anyone.

Myeloma
www.myeloma.org
Truly international site, with information on new treatments and own magazine; style, a bit formal.

Oral
www.dentalhealth.org
Information on oral cancers and treatment available in the UK from the British Dental Health Foundation.

Ovarian
www.ovarian.org
(US site). Information, help and clinical trials.

Pancreatic
www.pancan.org
(US site). Help for patients and their families.

Prostate
www.prostate.org.uk
Bright lively site with information, help, and chat lines and message boards. Order leaflets and info packs on-line. Excellent.

5. Clinical Trials

European Clinical Trials
www.EORTC.be
Monitors clinical trials, the development of new drugs, and other innovative approaches to improve the standard of cancer treatment in Europe.

Worldwide
www.nci.nih.gor
American top site for clinical trials.

APPENDIX III

A selection of books you might read:

Your Body's Energy — Emma Mitchell
Chakra Healing — Liz Simpson
Ayurvedic Home Remedies — Vasant Lad
Natural Detox — Marie Farquharson
Fit for Life — Marilyn Diamond
Instant Calm — Paul Wilson
The Road Less Travelled — M Scott Peck
Take Time for Your Life — Cheryl Richardson
Vibrational Medicine — Dr Richard Gerber
Food, Your Miracle Medicine — Jean Carter
Ageless Body, Timeless Mind — Deepak Chopra
Your Life in Your Hands — Professor Jane Plant
The Cancer Prevention Diet — Dr Rosie Daniels
Stopping the Clock — Dr Ronald Klatz and Dr Robert Goldman

The Vitamin Bible — Earl Mindell
Foods That Fight Pain — Dr Neal Barnard
Hands of Light — Barbara Ann Brennan
The Safe Shopper's Bible — David Steinman and Samuel Epstein
A Cancer Battle Plan Sourcebook — Dave Frahm

APPENDIX IV

Liver Cleanse / Gallstone Flush

Ingredients:
$^1/_2$ cup extra virgin olive oil
1 very big grapefruit (providing $^3/_4$ cup of juice)
4 tablespoons of Epsom Salts
3 cup of water
Ornithine tablets.

Preparation:
Set aside three days.

Day 1:
Eat a no-fat breakfast; and lunch.
Eat and drink nothing after 2.00 pm.
Mix the Epsom Salts in the water (easier if water is warm), then cool.

6.00 pm	Drink a quarter of this liquid.
8.00 pm	Drink a further quarter of the liquid
10.00 pm	Mix the olive oil and pulp-free grapefruit juice and shake vigorously.
	Drink the liquid through a straw before 10.15 pm.
	Take four Ornithine tablets to help you sleep.
	Retire immediately and massage your stomach.
	Focus your mind on your liver and imagine the toxins leaving it, along with the stones.
	Sleep.

Day 2:
Upon waking and not before 7.00 am take the third quarter of the Epsom salts mix. Two hours later take the last quarter.

Expect diarrhoea for two days; don't eat before lunch time on day two and keep food to salads and fruit, plus baked potatoes for days two and three.

You may need to repeat this treatment after a few weeks. 2000–3000 small stones may be passed.

Please note – This recipe is derived from William Kelley's cancer treatment. It has thousands of testimonials, none report pain, only success; but nobody at Health Issues has any first hand experience of it. We are merely **told** it works!

To order more copies of this book

Tel: 44(0)1280 815166
Fax: 44(0)1280 824655
Email: enquiries@iconmag.co.uk

For essential news, reviews and breakthroughs in cancer prevention and cure –

Take out a subscription to our monthly magazine *Icon*

tel: 44(0)1280 815166

For forthcoming books on everything you need to know about the specific cancers; or on 'eating to beat cancer' with diet tips, good foods and recipes

Tel: 44(0)1280 815166
Fax: 44(0)1280 824655
Email: enquiries@iconmag.co.uk